CANNABIS FOR LYME DISEASE AND RELATED CONDITIONS

Scientific Basis and Anecdotal Evidence for Medicinal Use

By Shelley M. White

DISCLAIMER

The author of this book is not a physician or doctor, and this book is not intended as medical advice. It is also not intended to prevent, diagnose, treat or cure disease. Instead, the book is intended only to share the author's research, as would an investigative journalist. The book is provided for informational and educational purposes only, not as treatment instructions for any disease.

Cannabis, or "medical marijuana," is not legal to purchase or use in some cities, states, and regions in the United States and other countries. Please do not purchase or use cannabis if it is not legal in your area. Obey your local laws. The laws and regulations in your city, state, region or country, should always be considered more accurate and authoritative than this book.

Lyme Disease is a dangerous disease and requires treatment by a licensed physician; this book is not a substitute for professional medical care. Do not begin any new treatment program without full consent and supervision from a licensed physician. If you have a medical problem, consult a doctor, not this book. If you are pregnant or breastfeeding, consult a physician before using any treatment.

Many of the treatments presented in this book are experimental and not FDA approved. Some of the book's content is speculative and theoretical. The author and publisher assume no liability or responsibility for any action taken by a reader of this book—use of this book is at your own risk. The statements in this book have not been evaluated by the FDA.

The author offers no guarantee that the treatments in this book are the best Lyme Disease therapies; instead, they were simply the treatments that the author found (through research and experience) to be worthy of writing about. Do not rely on this book as the final word in Lyme disease treatment.

For all who respect the intelligence of plants, for those who stood by me when I ventured into unknown territory to treat myself using unconventional methods, and most importantly for my mother and father for teaching me that it is more important to expose the truth than it is to be accepted by society. You are the reason I continued to push through the dark nights that begged me to give up. You are the reason I am able to sit here today and write these words. Simply saying "thank you" could never be enough.

CONTENTS

Chapter 5

Chapter 6

PART TWO: USING CANNABIS TO REDUCE THE SYMPTOMS OF LYME DISEASE AND RELATED CONDITIONS

Chapter 7

Chapter 8

Chapter 9

Chapter 10

Foreword

BY JULIE MCINTYRE, CLINICAL HERBALIST

Lyme disease is a pathogen of sophisticated stealthiness, meaning the spirochete bacteria that causes Lyme disease is able to sequester itself inside host cells to avoid the immune system's detection. These bacteria affect a variety of body organs, tissues, cells, and glands. The symptoms they create in the body have led to calling Lyme disease the "great imitator" for it mimics MS, fibromyalgia, chronic fatigue syndrome, Parkinson's, Alzheimer's, heart disease, irritable bowel syndrome, metabolic diseases and psychotic episodes.

Because of the stealth nature and intelligence of the organisms, we necessarily must approach healing Lyme disease using treatments that are not common in the way we have been taught to think about treating bacterial infections. (I mean, it's just a *bacterium*.) The world is not the same as it was when penicillin was developed. We now see the effects of the mistakes that were made then with overuse of antibiotics and the resultant antibiotic resistant bacteria. Many of those mistakes were due to hubris.

What we know now is that bacteria are extremely intelligent and adaptable. They communicate with each other over long distances sharing information about antibiotic resistance (a phenomenon known as "quorum sensing"). They seem always to be one step ahead of research. The fact that microbes can bring us to our knees and humble us in ways we dare not imagine in our healthiest moments ought to be the end of thinking we are the smartest species at the top of the food chain. If you doubt this, recall the last time you had strep throat, the flu or a urinary tract infection.

Bacteria are the oldest forms of life on Earth; three billion years old. They have survived because of their level of intelligence and adaptability. They have learned to alter their structures and respond to substances they come in contact with and rather quickly.

They have a variety of structures called efflux pumps that act as a type of sump pump. When a substance assaults the cell membrane the bacteria essentially pumps it back out. But it is not random. Bacteria have created a wide range of pump types to protect themselves from all manner of antimicrobial substances.

What makes plant medicines (herbal antibiotics) elegantly effective agents to treat antibiotic resistant bacteria is that plants, in order to survive, are in a constant state of analyzing their environment and altering their chemical compounds to address threats to their health whether it is bacterial, viral or insect. Essentially, they are their own physicians. Not only do plant medicines have antibacterial actions, they have complex chemical constituents making them multi-system agents of healing. Cannabis is a perfect example. It has over 700 broadly active constituents making it an intelligent choice for reducing inflammation, relieving pain, alleviating insomnia and soothing anxiety.

Humans, and many other species, are hard wired with an endo-cannabinoid system throughout the brain and body thus making the use of marijuana a logical and intelligent choice of medicine. The endocannabinoid system is composed of neuromodulatory lipids and their receptors. Unique to the cannabis plant alone are cannabinoids, specific constituents that bind to the body's endocannabinoid receptors, and as Shelley notes in this book, "... regulate physiological processes such as appetite, pain interpre-tation, memory, and mood." Cannabinoids modulate the release of neurotransmitters such as GABA, 5HTP, glutamate, acetyl-choline, noradrenalin, and dopamine from a number of central nervous system structures.

Parents desperate for options to help their children often find that medical marijuana is the key to giving their children with seizure disorders a chance at a normal life. There is a despera-tion and fierceness in people who themselves (or their children) have a symptom picture that is debilitating. Weeks and years of insomnia or epilepsy can cause one to not care about laws banning the use of a natural substance that could bring sleep or relief. Those suffering from the symptoms of Lyme disease often find tremendous relief from using cannabis, dramatically reducing temporal lobe seizures as well as insomnia, neuropath-ic pain, lack of appetite, joint pain, and muscular pain.

Nevertheless, this tremendously effective medicine has suffered decades of prohibition. Until 1998 when California became the first state to legalize marijuana for medical use. Slowly, but with increasing regularity, the herb is seeing more acceptance.

Sanjay Gupta, M.D., CNN's Chief Medical Correspondent, for example, has publicly announced his backing of marijuana for medical use years after he made a blanket statement condemning it. Gupta has since apologized for his statements saying he didn't look hard enough or far enough, nor did he look at the research coming out of the smaller labs.

> *I mistakenly believed the Drug Enforcement Agency listed marijuana as a schedule 1 substance based on sound scientific proof. Surely, they must have quality reasoning as to why marijuana is in the category of the most dangerous drugs that have "no accepted medical use and a high potential for abuse."*

> *They didn't have the science to support that claim, and I now know that when it comes to marijuana neither of those things are true. It doesn't have a high potential for abuse, and there are very legitimate medical applications. In fact, sometimes marijuana is the only thing that works.*

He goes on to say,

> *We have been terribly and systematically misled for nearly 70 years in the United States, and I apologize for my own role in that.* [A]

I take hope in this rare, intelligent, even socially unacceptable, conversion regarding the decriminalization and legalization of marijuana. As well as the growing number of states making medical marijuana legal. Simply, the reality that CBD oil from hemp that is legal in every state (and orderable through the internet) gives rise to hope and the potential for marijuana to become widely and easily available. Marijuana has a legitimate place in the materia medica and pharmacopoeia as a real and viable herbal remedy.

As a society we have a responsibility to those who are ill to make every possible avenue to healing available to them. Anything less is cruelty. Unfortunately, the deplorable situation with cannabis acceptance is all too often mirrored in medical and societal approaches to Lyme disease.

As a clinical herbalist I hear or read stories every day from my clients that cause me to shake my head in shame of our Western, industrial, first world medical system. I'm outraged on behalf of my clients for the humiliation, lack of care and lack of time devoted to their patient needs. Every week if not every day I hear stories of physicians denying that Lyme disease exists in their state or they blame the patient for "faking symptoms" to get attention, or they refer their patients for psychiatric counseling. The stories are endless and horrific in the ramifications they have on people trying to find help in the midst of devastating illness and debilitating pain. In a research abstract entitled *Bullying Borrelia: when the culture of science is under attack*, the authors state the following:

> *Although Lyme disease responds to short courses of antibiotics, tick-borne Borrelia Burgdorferi has been advanced by some as a frequent explanation for medically unexplained symptoms... Perhaps due to the lack of supportive data, proponents of this theory have developed their own meetings, literature, activist groups, and substantial internet activities to advance their views ... While neither logical nor evidence-based, 'chronic Lyme disease' harnesses corrosive energies that taint modern medicine and society.* [B]

Many researchers and clinicians find such statements to be unscientific and counterproductive. For example, Christian Perronne, MD, PhD, is a Professor of Infectious and Tropical Diseases at the Faculty of Medicine Ile-de-France Ouest, and President of the

French Federation of Infectiology (FFI). He is also Vice-President of the European Advisory Group of Experts on Immunization at the World Health Organization, and is the author or co-author of 218 scientific publications.

In the May, 2012 edition of *The Lancet Infectious Diseases* (volume 12), Dr. Perronne made the following statements (reprinted with permission):

> *Paul Auwaerter and colleagues compare some Lyme disease activists who use non-evidence-based arguments with anti-HIV or antivaccination extremists. Their Personal View shows that unscientific thinking and malpractice occur in many specialties. Such a focus has unfortunately resulted in suppression of legitimate and necessary scientific debate about the management of syndromes of unclear aetiology, which sometimes occur after a previously proven episode of Lyme disease or tick bites. Public health recommendations should rely on strong evidence-based data and not on expert opinion, as Lee and Vielmeyer's review of the Infectious Disease Society of America guidelines shows is the case with Lyme disease.*

> *Recommended serological tests for Lyme disease vary greatly in sensitivity. Since no reliable reference standard exists—such as a specific clinical score, culture, or PCR—the cut-off levels of such tests are decided with healthy donors and calculated arbitrarily. Several studies have shown that seronegative Lyme disease cases can be proved with culture or PCR. Seronegative patients have been included as Lyme disease cases in a major clinical trial.*

> *Another difficulty is that, although many variants and new species of Borrelia are regularly discovered, most*

commercial tests rely on the original Massachusetts B31 isolate of Borrelia burgdorferi, used since 1982. However, Scottish experts were able to improve the sensitivity of their tests with local strains of Borrelia spp. In Brazil, a Lyme-like syndrome has also been described that is due to a non-cultivable spirochete—not a Borrelia species—and is therefore undetected by current serological tests.

Additionally, peer-reviewed studies show that other bacterial, viral, or parasitic infections might contribute to syndromes associated with Lyme disease or its mimics. Microbial involvement is being actively investigated in other well known but poorly understood conditions. For example, the possible role of spirochetes, including B. burgdorferi, has become the subject of research into the pathophysiology of Alzheimer's disease.

Syndromes without a clear cause or objective evidence should no longer be called chronic Lyme disease. These syndromes are probably caused by several factors; therefore, both infectious and non-infectious aetiologies should be considered. To limit the debate to Lyme disease alone is highly unproductive, because this disease is unlikely to be the universal explanation of our patients' persisting ailments. These syndromes with possible microbial involvement should be investigated with the best available tests and with a fresh and open-minded scientific approach.[c]

There are the few and rare physicians who care enough and are brave enough to think outside the box of their allopathic training and treatment limitations for alternative options and hope, often risking their license to do so. One of the things they have in common is that they *listen* to their patients.

I have felt from my earliest days of treating people with Lyme disease and related conditions that my clients are my greatest teachers. They are the best researched, most intelligent, brave and tenacious group of people I have ever worked with.

They keep me humble. They have their pulse on the latest research, latest treatments, and newest practitioners. They think and live outside normal boundaries of thinking and living. People who are chronically ill, afraid, desperate for help and feel alone are willing to try about anything if there is a chance it will help them regain health. Coming from this pool of people, innovating on medicines and out-of-the-box treatments, we find the healing properties and symptom-reducing actions of medical marijuana.

Many people with Lyme disease first begin by looking for treatments inside the allopathic community. They find sooner or later, (and often after spending tens of thousands of dollars on antibiotic treatment) that the old ways of treating bacterial infections are not working; that healing inside the established system does not work for a very large segment of the Lyme community. That system is, unfortunately, wrought with archaic beliefs and limited treatment options. Those who work within the system are finding that they themselves are limited, not only by the resources available to them, but also by the constraints of their licensure requirements, and most importantly, by their training, which has limited them to see only what they have been trained to see. One of these limits is their rather archaic view of plant medicines.

Plant medicines have complex chemical constituents that can sophisticatedly modulate our body's physical, chemical and electrical systems. They help our bodies remember how to be well. And they often open us up to other views of reality. This way of seeing and the alterations plants cause in our awareness are part of the reasons marijuana has been illegal for seventy years.

My own personal journey is, I suppose, not all that different than many Lyme patients and medical physicians.

In 1982 Lyme disease was far removed from my daily thoughts, as it still was to the news reports and in personal conversations. I remember hearing rumblings of Lyme disease later in that decade; still there was a feeling of immunity in those of us who heard rumors of it. It was not as if any of us could catch it.

Lyme only began to become real to me while enrolled in an EMT training course. One of the required classes was "How to keep oneself safe while out on an ambulance call." The woman teaching the class was passionately and skillfully telling a story of first responders and paramedics becoming infected with Lyme disease while responding to car accidents and roll-overs in grassy ditches. I stopped breathing and moving while the horror of the symptom description, and the rapidly declining health and functionality of those who had become infected, washed through my brain like a tsunami. In that instant the world became a much smaller place for me.

I didn't know then that my destiny was already pulling me along, insisting I take my place in the midst of one of the fastest growing bacterial epidemics of the modern era.

The instructor painted a graphic picture for me and the years since have filled in the picture considerably. I have now heard thousands of stories of Lyme disease...from the initial bite, to years and decades of declining health, debilitating symptoms, and unsuccessful attempts at getting an accurate diagnosis and effective treatment. Distressingly, after years of increasing symptoms, insomnia, psychosis and pain, many people suffering from Lyme disease find they must endure further suffering in the form of ridicule, abandonment, and financial devastation. They lose friends, marriages and homes.

People with Lyme disease, and/or coinfections, are some of the bravest people I have met. Many of them have traveled alone into the darkness of the illness and in the process, ultimately, found others like themselves. Whole communities have grown up around Lyme disease that address the illness, symptoms, protocols, experiences with physicians and alternative practitioners and treatments. This is a demographic of the world population that is willing to think outside of the box primarily because their experiences inside the rules of conduct of seeking medical help have not served them and in many instances caused damage despite the medical dictum: *First, do no harm.*

Once one has walked the arduous, terrifying and lonely journey a chronic illness is, the person emerging from the tangled forest of illness is not the same as the one who entered. Chronic illness has a function and that is to change us.

Once we have had the experience of a plant saving our life we are never the same again. The fact of a plant or plants saving our lives, alleviating our suffering, raising our spirit and level of hope changes our beliefs about reality and what we have been told. We have been forced by circumstances and events to re-examine our beliefs and ideas about how the world is made up. We question what we thought was reality, the rules we were told to obey and the authorities who wrote them.

All throughout life, people adapt and make concessions to fit into the world of work and productivity, the choices of which cause disturbing ripples in the soul. More often than not, in the midst of an illness crisis when one is most vulnerable, newer insight into the life being lived occurs. Many begin to follow the inclinations of long ago childhood dreams. They remember they've always wanted to become a dancer, pianist, writer. Sometimes the dream that emerges is to become an herbalist.

These are those who experienced plants healing them by bringing strength back to limbs that began to fail, sleep for the first time in years, or improved memory and an end to Lyme induced psychosis. Sometimes the healing that occurs stops what the person was doing and rekindles the fires of what they were meant to be all along. And there are many who found themselves about to fall off the edge into the abyss when unexpectedly, wild green tendrils reached out to clasp their wrist. They were pulled back to solid ground, giving them courage and endurance to face another day.

In the pages of this book you'll find easy-to-read scientific research on the mechanisms and actions of medical marijuana and how these constituents affect individual symptoms of Lyme disease. The bookends holding together and supporting the scientific research are composed of the story of one woman's journey, of her life being turned inside out from a debilitating disease and her discovery of the plant that healed her. In the midst of illness and her discovery of the plant that companioned her, she found herself. Ultimately, each of us must find our own truth, our own path of healing. I pray that we each have the freedom to do just that. Shelley's book is a welcome and needed addition to that freedom.

Julie McIntyre, Clinical Herbalist

References

A. Gupta, Sanjay, CNN.com 8/8/2013

B. Auwaerter PG; Melia MT; *Bullying Borrelia: when the culture of science is under attack,* PubMed 2012:123:79-89, PMID: 23303970. Trans Am Clin Climatol Assoc. 2012; 123: 79–90

C. Reprinted from *The Lancet Infectious Diseases*, Volume 12, Christian Perronne, Lyme disease antiscience, pages 361-362, 2012, with permission from Elsevier / The Lancet.

Preface

Tired of lingering on the brink where death and life collide, I scanned my room at 3:00 A.M. for something I could use to kill myself to no avail. Rolling over in the bed which I had spent 90% of the past two years of my life in, my eyes fell on the stealthy sack of marijuana next to my bed and only one thought went through my head, *"screw it. I'm going to get high out of my mind."*

As it would turn out, this seemingly self-destructive thought was my ticket in disguise to life. Instead of smoking my brains out, as I originally intended to do, I unknowingly took the first step towards reclaiming it when I began loading my pipe. Little did I know, the very moments I was contemplating suicide were the ones that gave me what I had so desperately been seeking—the opportunity to once again feel alive.

Contrary to popular belief, the thoughts of those under the influence of cannabis are not "dumb." Well, sometimes they are, but not always. Society views a person who is high as someone whose thinking is "impaired." That night begs me to ask the question of whose thinking is truly impaired, though, because after countless hits of weed my doors of perception opened and I saw things clearer than I had in years. My usually irrational, frantic thoughts which constantly ran a race with no finish line transmuted into rational, steady ones working in synchronicity with one another to methodically create their own destiny.

"If all herbs are useful, and there are over seven-hundred known healing components in cannabis, why not find out what it does when used to treat Lyme disease?" was the final thought that went through my head before I blindly ventured into the dark waters of the unknown without a trace of hesitation. You must understand, though, that that final thought in no way implied I would play it safe but that I would intentionally play it as dangerous as humanly possible and consume ungodly amounts of cannabis on a consistent basis. History can attest to the fact that the moments you have nothing to lose, the moments you have no attachments to or in life, are ironically the exact moments when you begin to open your eyes and become vibrantly alive.

To say the controversy regarding medicinal use of cannabis was of little concern to me at this point would be an understatement, it was of absolutely no concern to me—except in the sense that I knew people would try and stop me. So, I let relatively no one in on my plan, and instead began executing it at full force. The results were magnificent. Within a few months, cannabis oil had done what years of antibiotics had failed to do. It had given me my life back, and I was once again driving, working, and hanging out with friends. High on the fact I had gotten my health back, I packed up and moved to a new state to work at a publishing company I greatly admired. I acted carelessly, failing to give my body enough time to recuperate before making such a move. Furthermore, I ceased taking cannabis oil altogether and did not stay on a maintenance dose as I had planned to, naively assuming

I was cured. These two acts played a major role in my inevitable relapse.

My relapse was so great that I was sure I would die of the feeling of defeat it ensued as opposed to Lyme disease itself. However, after a few months of wallowing in self-pity, I worked up the courage to once again begin taking a homemade, gentle cannabis oil recipe in large amounts. Throughout the day, I would take doses every few hours, as doing so seemed to lessen the severity of my symptoms. Please note, though, that I did experience intense Herxheimer reactions at night when I took larger doses. The oil, combined with a few other revelations in my health mystery, successfully helped bring me back to life a second time. I do not feel comfortable calling cannabis oil a "cure" for Lyme disease, as the subject of whether or not it is possible to fully cure advanced cases of Lyme disease is still a heated debate in the medical and Lyme community alike due to the elusive nature of bacteria. I do, however, feel comfortable saying that cannabis oil greatly reduced the severity of my symptom picture and improved my quality of life while going through Lyme treatment. I also personally feel that cannabis oil significantly speeds up the process of healing.

After the first time I hit remission with the help of cannabis, I wrote an article on my experience and quickly published it online on my way out the door one day. Little did I know, it would spark a collective movement in the Lyme community, fueled by each individual's fury to heal at all costs—a fury I know all too well. I would spend hours answering emails from people with questions about treating their Lyme disease with cannabis, and still failed to answer all the questions pouring into my inbox. Unable to answer all of the emails I was receiving, and feeling as if I was not giving the amount of attention deserved to the ones I did answer, left me feeling hopeless and frustrated. How could

I help everyone all at once? I am hoping this book answers that question. Please remember, I am not a medical doctor, and the information I provide represents my own personal experiences and opinions. Please consult a licensed doctor before making any treatment decisions.

While I have received innumerable supportive emails regarding my decision to treat myself with cannabis oil, which I am deeply grateful for, I have also received emails filled with hatred and criticism. This has opened my eyes to one of the most profound truths my journey to regain my health has taught me: people fear most what they do not understand. So, with that in mind, I composed the following pages for those who wish to expand their understanding of the healing powers of cannabis; both for Lyme disease and related conditions.

I am well aware that at the same time as I write these words, a war long ago waged on cannabis continues to rage on. My intentions in writing this book are not to convince anyone of anything or to soothe the conflict over cannabis in any way. Rather, my intentions are to offer factual evidence from my own personal accounts accompanied with in depth research for those interested in expanding their knowledge on the medicinal properties of cannabis relevant to the treatment of Lyme disease and related conditions.

PART ONE:

FUNDAMENTAL PRINCIPLES OF USING CANNABIS TO TREAT LYME AND RELATED CONDITIONS

Chapter 1

CANNABIS AS A BACTERICIDAL AGENT AND AS A TOOL FOR SYMPTOM MANAGEMENT

D ue to the steady emergence and continued increase of drug resistant bacteria, new classes of antibacterial agents are urgently needed. As history shows, synthetic, man-made antibacterial agents lack the ability to effectively eradicate the ever evolving bacteria in our ecosystem once they successfully deem human bodies as their hosts. Initially effective antibiotics are rendered relatively useless over time. For example, resistance to the class of antibacterials most commonly used to treat E. coli induced urinary tract infections, fluoroquinolones, exists worldwide. When first introduced in the 1980s, there was virtually no bacterial resistance to fluoroquinolones.[1] The difference in the characteristics of present day bacteria, such as spirochetes, is unparalleled in nature compared to the characteristics they displayed as little as five years ago. On the contrary, the pharmaceuticals used to treat them have remained very much the same. We have failed to evolve in intelligence at a rate proportional to that of bacteria, resulting in the mass difficulties we now face in treating bacterial infections such as Lyme disease and related conditions.

We have made the dire, self-destructive mistake of assuming bacteria are unintelligent organisms. In doing so, bacteria have superseded us and learned to adapt and evolve in ways enabling them to evade the threat of antibiotics and other pharmaceuticals commonly used to treat them. An astounding amount of evidence points towards a desperate need for the discovery and/or invention of new classes of antibacterial agents, yet the number of antibacterials being released continues to drop. From 1983-1987, approximately 16 new antibacterials were approved by the FDA, while under five have been approved since 2008. Many pharmaceutical companies have ceased research and development of antibacterial drugs, lending to the sharp decline of new antibacterials released in the past 30 years. Coincidentally, the past 30 years fall grotesquely in alignment with the time period in which spirochetes have rapidly evolved into a dangerously aggressive species of bacteria. Although plants such as cannabis are equipped with secondary metabolites that display antibacterial qualities potent enough to effectively target, reach, and treat drug resistant bacteria, plants in general still remain markedly unexploited antimicrobial agents. This notion is highly insulting to the intelligence of the human mind, yet nonetheless holds great validity.

Cannabis as a Bactericide

Research indicates that cannabis is an excellent and effective bactericide, meaning it is able to destroy or inhibit the growth of bacteria, due to its impeccably composed chemical profile. Its compounds are able to bypass the healing powers, or lack thereof, of man-made bactericides like antibiotics in order to effectively kill drug resistant bacteria or "superbugs." Compounds in cannabis known as cannabinoids, for example, appear to go unscathed by mechanisms typically used by bacteria to evade antibiotics. For example, cannabinoids effectively combat the drug resistant type of staph known as methicillin-resistant *Staphylococcus aureus* (MRSA).[2]

In regards to Lyme disease, bacterial die-off from cannabis is most noticeable when it is taken in relatively high amounts (exact amounts vary depending on form of use, as we will discuss later), often sparking a "Jarisch-Herxheimer Reaction," which is an exacerbation of symptoms also informally referred to as a "Herxheimer Reaction," "Herx," or "Herxing." A Herxheimer Reaction is instigated when dying bacteria release their endotoxins into the bloodstream and tissues faster than the body can successfully expel them from its system, prompting an excessive inflammatory response. Simply put, toxins flood the body at a rate not proportional to the body's ability to comfortably detox them, causing an overload of toxins in the body, thus increasing inflammation and worsening symptoms. A lessening, to some degree, of symptom severity gradually becomes apparent as endotoxins released from the bacterial die-off are adequately removed from the body system, and the Herxheimer Reaction subsides.

Many are afraid of the mental impairment or "high" cannabis often causes, lending to the current craze over CBD oils, which contain little if any traces of the psychoactive ingredient THC (tetrahydrocannabinol). However, pure cannabis, as opposed to CBD oil, is likely to be more effective as a bactericide. CBD oil consists of cannabidiol, only one of five major cannabinoids found in cannabis that displays potent activity in treating drug resistant strains of bacteria. Research has shown four other cannabinoids—cannabichromene, cannabigerol, tetrahydro-cannabinol, and cannabinol—display significant antibacterial properties as well. So, while it is true that CBD oil is beneficial for treating certain infections and easing symptoms of certain conditions, it is also true that the whole form of the herb is potentially four times as potent as an antibacterial agent.

Cannabinoids are not the only healing compounds in cannabis, though. Also of importance are the terpenoids and flavonoids found in cannabis. Terpenoids, which are also found in mammals where they serve as vehicles to expel parasites, tend to have a synergistic effect with cannabinoids and increase their efficiency as bactericidal agents. Terpenoids in cannabis help counteract THC-induced anxiety and lend to its effectiveness at relieving symptoms of depression, pain, brain inflammation, joint inflammation, addiction, and epilepsy. The flavonoids in cannabis are called cannaflavins. Pharmacological activities of cannaflavins are shown to be up to thirty times more effective at reducing inflammation than aspirin. On a biochemical level, cannaflavins inhibit enzymatic processes, interact with estrogen receptors, and act as powerful antioxidants.

Argument Against Using Cannabis as an Antibacterial Agent

Paradoxically, some studies have linked cannabis use to an increase in opportunistic infections and an interference with nitric oxide production from macrophages in the pulmonary system, thereby impairing defense mechanisms against pathogens in the respiratory system.[3] These studies have understandably prompted many to close their minds to considering the impressively vast array of life changing and/or life saving healing properties of cannabis.

It is worth noting that, just like cannabis, pharmaceuticals with potential benefits can also prove harmful—especially when large doses are steadily taken for an extended amount of time. Unlike cannabis, pharmaceuticals can prove lethal if used incorrectly—to date, I am not aware of a single death directly resulting from cannabis use. Also worth noting is that heavy use of any substance, whether it be cannabis, pharmaceuticals, or anything else, often manifests as a result of an individual's inability to cope with overwhelming depression or stress. Individuals who are depressed or stressed already have significantly weaker immune systems than emotionally stable individuals, regardless of cannabis or any other substances, meaning their susceptibility to contracting opportunistic infections was already elevated to begin with. It is also important to consider that most of these studies were conducted on individuals who smoke cannabis, as opposed to those who use other methods of consumption. Smoking it will temporarily impair the immune system because of possible carcinogens and toxins on the plant itself, and the combustion of these harmful components from the raw plant material due to the high temperature at which it is burned.

The solution to the immunosuppressant effects from interference of nitric oxide production in the pulmonary system caused by smoking cannabis truly is quite simple. Do not smoke it. Opt for other methods of use, such as oils, vaporizing or edibles. Most importantly, use logic and reasoning when taking into consideration the possible medicinal benefits you or someone you know may reap from cannabis use.

Dosing Considerations When Utilizing Cannabis as a Bactericide

Upon initial consideration of using cannabis to treat Lyme disease and Lyme disease co-infections, the majority of your preconceived notions regarding its medicinal uses for other illnesses may need to be dropped, as other illnesses tend to be entirely different in nature than Lyme disease and Lyme disease co-infections. Just the same, no two cases of Lyme disease are alike; a fact which only serves to further complicate matters. There are countless strains of cannabis, each with their own possible pros and cons, with the existence of these pros and cons being heavily situation dependent. The dosage which is correct for you may not work for another person with Lyme disease and vice versa. The dosing guidelines for using cannabis oil to treat cancer, for example, cannot be looked at with validity in relation to treating Lyme disease. Although a certain amount of cannabis may prove beneficial and harmless to a cancer patient, a person with Lyme disease who takes the same amount without first slowly working their way up to it may experience an extreme Herxheimer Reaction. When treating yourself with cannabis for Lyme disease, refrain from automatically adopting the dosing guidelines of someone else, with or without Lyme disease, as an indicator of how much you should take. Rather, start at the lowest possible dose you can, which will vary depending on what form you are consuming it in—i.e. if you are using a vaporizer, a single, quick inhalation may be the lowest dose you can start at. If you are using oil, one drop under the tongue may be the lowest starting dose (or you may even choose to dilute a drop of oil in water and then consume only part of the water solution to effectively take a fraction of a drop). Please remember, though, that I am not a medical doctor, and therefore I do not intend for this book to be used as dosing instructions; instead, please consult with your physician before beginning any new treatments.

Also, please only use cannabis if it is legal in your location; do not break any applicable laws.

Considering cannabis is bactericidal and can cause a Herxheimer Reaction, you must stay mindful of how your body responds to it, using its responses as clues to shape the correct dosing guidelines for your specific case. Start by ingesting the lowest amount of cannabis possible and slowly work your way up, using your body's reactions as clues as to whether you should continue increasing your dosage. If symptoms worsen to an intolerable degree when you increase your dose, decrease your dose to the amount you were previously taking. Once again, to reiterate, the correct amount of cannabis to use when treating Lyme disease varies per person, unlike other illnesses which have an established approximate dosing baseline. Every case of Lyme disease varies significantly. The way you respond to a specific amount or strain of cannabis may differ greatly from the way another person with Lyme disease responds to the same two factors, depending on variables such as which co-infections each of you may or may not be infected with, and to what extent you may or may not be infected with them.

Since cannabis use can cause a Herxheimer Reaction from bacterial die-off, it is important to implement detoxification methods into your treatment protocol to assist your body in ridding itself of toxins in order to lessen the severity of your symptoms and speed up the rate at which you heal. If you have a MTHFR gene mutation, which is not uncommon in patients with chronic and persistent Lyme disease, then it is especially important to employ rigorous and strict detoxification methods into your protocol. MTHFR is the gene that administers instructions to the methylenetetrahydrofolate reductase (MTHFR) enzyme, which is an enzyme that plays a role in the body's methylation process. When an MTHFR gene malfunctions, methylation pathways are blocked and natural detoxification becomes extremely challenging for the body. In other words, detox pathways are sealed shut, allowing toxins to pile up in the body. To ensure this does not happen, adamantly detox on a steady, daily basis. For many, implementing various methods of detox is necessary.

Reducing Your Symptom Picture with Cannabis

Aside from working as a bactericide, cannabis also possesses the power to significantly reduce your overall symptom picture throughout the duration of treatment. When used for symptom picture reduction, dosing is much lower than it is when used for bactericidal purposes, as larger doses may spark a bacterial die-off that exacerbates symptoms. Of course, the extent to which it does or does not alleviate symptom severity has to do with various factors, such as the amount of cannabis you use, the strain you use, and the form you take it in (i.e. oils, smoking, vaporizing, or edibles). Part one of this book was created to better equip you with information on these subjects. Part two was created with the intent of helping you develop an understanding of which of your symptoms cannabis may alleviate and how it may do so, enabling you to target your worst symptoms to increase your quality of life during treatment. In combination, both parts of this book are meant to give you the tools to formulate an outline for the best way to treat your specific case.

Dosing Considerations When Using Cannabis for Symptom Management

When used in relatively small amounts, cannabis can also work to lessen the severity of your symptoms. When finding the correct dosing levels of cannabis for symptom maintenance, you will have to undergo the same trial and error process as you did when finding a dose of cannabis that kills off bacteria at a rate which you can comfortably handle. Start with a miniscule amount and work your way up, slowly increasing your dose according to your body's reaction to the herb. Personally, I was partial towards using cannabis as a bactericide at night and as a tool for symptom relief during the day, meaning I took considerably larger amounts at night than I did during the day. In doing so, I was neither impaired by the substance or the effects of a Herxheimer Reaction during the day and was able to live a higher quality of life. For information on available cannabis products and consumption options, refer to chapter four.

Remember to consult a physician prior to using cannabis or any other treatment. I am a Lyme patient and researcher, not a doctor, so the dosing information here represents my opinion and experience only.

Chapter 2

CHEMICAL CONSTITUENTS OF CANNABIS

Developing an understanding of the chemical constituents of cannabis is of immense importance for anyone wishing to comprehend the science behind the plant's medicinal benefits. A large variety of chemical compounds have been identified in cannabis, totaling over 700 to date. While many of these compounds are found in other plant species as well, some are unique to the cannabis plant alone, such as cannabinoids. Other identified chemical constituents in cannabis include terpenes, proteins, flavonoids, amino acids, carbohydrates, fatty acids, non-cannabinoid phenols, ketones, aldehydes, esters, lactones, vitamin K, essential elements, minerals, and more. Of all of the chemical constituents found in cannabis, cannabinoids, terpenes, and flavonoids possess the most known health benefits.

Cannabinoids and other cannabis constituents found in cannabis instigate a wide array of effects in the human body system primarily by binding to receptor sites in cell walls throughout various locations in the body. This is an exemplary demonstration of the deeply meaningful, close, and valuable relationship between mankind and cannabis. Perhaps worth consideration is this: yes, harmful effects of cannabis use have been reported *mostly in cases where it was used in excess, similar to virtually all prescription medications, over the counter medications, herbal products, supplements, and basically anything else in the world that may have harmful consequences when used in excess, including things as seemingly harmless as water or air.*

Understanding the Endocannabinoid System

Many of the body's interactions with cannabis take place within the body's endocannabinoid system. The endocannabinoid system is located throughout the brain and body, and is composed of neuromodulatory lipids and their receptors. Cannabinoids, for example, interact with the endocannabinoid system to modulate important bodily functions that determine how an individual moves, reacts, and feels both physically and mentally. Cannabinoids also bind to receptors in the body's endocannabinoid system to regulate physiological processes such as appetite, pain interpretation, memory, and mood—and so much more, as you will soon find out. Research has found an underlying clinical endocannabinoid deficiency may be the root cause of conditions like chronic migraines, fibromyalgia, and irritable bowel syndrome, and cannabinoids may be a suitable treatment option for these conditions.[1]

Anandamide (AEA)

Serving as one of the most well-known endocannabinoids in the human body, AEA is produced by the body and regulates the central nervous system and immune system—mechanisms of extreme importance in those with Lyme disease who tend to have overactive central nervous systems and compromised immune systems. When functioning properly, AEA is a superb immunomodulator. It keeps the immune system strong enough to ward off infection, while simultaneously preventing it from becoming so strong it induces an adverse reaction in which the body's own immune system attacks itself. Immunomodulators are crucial for properly regulating malfunctioning immune systems. Cannabinoids interact with AEA in the endocannabinoid system to restore the body's ability to serve as its own immunomodulator. AEA also regulates memory functioning, appetite, sleep cycles, and sensations such as pleasure and pain.

While obtaining optimal functioning in all of these areas is obviously helpful to fully heal, attempting to do so can prove a daunting task. So, it may be helpful to tackle one problematic area at a time, as opposed to trying to improve all areas at once. One of the most important challenges to first focus on is achieving restoration and maintenance of a healthy sleep cycle. Doing so is of extreme importance when trying to heal, as many with Lyme disease and related conditions suffer from insomnia. When adequate sleep is not achieved, cells are unable to repair themselves and detoxification processes become impaired. The body detoxes more between the hours of 11:00 PM. and 3:00 A.M. than at any other time, making it absolutely paramount to place tremendous effort towards habitually falling asleep before 11:00 P.M. every night. When your sleep schedule is off, everything is off, and symptoms significantly increase in severity. The chapter on Insomnia in part two of this book will further discuss the role cannabis plays in combating sleep problems.

CB1 Receptors

CB1 Receptors are cannabinoid receptors primarily found throughout parts of the endocannabinoid system located in the brain, as well as in the female and male reproductive systems. Despite skeptics voicing concerns that cannabinoids lead to heart damage, heart disease, heart failure, and respiratory problems, CB1 receptors are found in areas of the brain stem responsible for regulating activities in the respiratory and cardiovascular systems. CB1 receptors, when bound with cannabinoids, are responsible for the euphoric and anticonvulsant properties of cannabis.

**Please note: Some research indicates that cannabis may have negative effects on the heart and cardiovascular system; this is a controversial area of research. Please consult your physician before using cannabis. Personally, I haven't seen convincing evidence that cannabis can negatively impact the heart.

CB2 Receptors

CB2 receptors are primarily scattered throughout parts of the endocannabinoid system located in the immune system, with the majority of them existing in the spleen. The relationship between CB2 receptors and cannabis accounts for much of the anti-inflammatory effects of cannabis. Cannabinoids such as THC act as agonists when they bind with cannabinoid receptors, such as CB2 receptors, by activating the receptors and instigating biological responses. CB2 agonists prompt the brain to release dopamine and serotonin, making them useful for treating inflammatory and neuropathic pain.

CB2 receptor agonists have therapeutic effects in those with neurodegenerative diseases, such as Alzheimer's disease, due to their ability to reduce brain inflammation.[2] This is also beneficial for those with encephalitis from Lyme disease or other conditions, in which individuals are prone to memory loss as a result of brain inflammation. Modulating CB2 receptors with agonists may also be the key for treating a plethora of other illnesses, as a variety of illnesses cause changes in CB2 receptor expressions, including cardiovascular, gastrointestinal, liver, kidney, psychiatric, bone, skin, lung and autoimmune diseases, as well as various forms of cancer.

Cannabinoids

Cannabinoids are the most well-known chemical constituents in cannabis, and they are more frequently and extensively researched than any other compound in cannabis. The medicinal qualities of cannabinoids stem from their ability to interact with the body's endocannabinoid system. Over 66 cannabinoids in cannabis have been identified. Some of the cannabinoids with known medicinal benefits include delta-9-tetrahydrocannabinol (THC), delta-9-tetrahydrocannabivarin (THCV), cannabidiol (CBD), cannabidiolic acid (CBDA), cannabichromene (CBC), cannabigerolic acid (CBGA), cannabigerol (CBG), and cannabinol (CBN).

As powerful anti-inflammatory agents, among other things, cannabinoids display many medicinal qualities with potential to prove beneficial in the treatment of Lyme disease, Lyme disease co-infections, and other ailments which manifest symptoms similar to these conditions. One of the most significant ways in which they may do so lies in their ability to suppress cytokine production—which there is a dangerously excessive amount of in Lyme disease and Lyme disease co-infections and which are responsible for the manifestation of a large majority of symptoms. Also of medicinal significance in regards to Lyme disease and associated conditions is the fact that cannabinoids promote induction of T-regulatory cells, which are cells that fight auto-immunity. The following are only some of the most extensively researched cannabinoids; there are many others.

Delta-9-tetrahydrocannabinol (THC)

Delta-9-tetrahydrocannabinol, more commonly known as THC, is one of the most universally recognized cannabinoids and is responsible for the psychoactive effects of cannabis. Some of the most popularly known medicinal uses of cannabis are attributable to THC, including its properties as an anti-inflammatory, anti-epileptic, anti-depressant, appetite stimulant, pain reliever, antiemetic (anti-nausea), and analgesic. THC can be beneficial for treating high blood pressure, glaucoma, and cancer. It may help improve cognitive functions by sharpening the mind and enhancing all sensory functions including sight, hearing, and sensitivity to colors. It inhibits vomiting by interacting with the 5-HT3A receptor, making it potentially useful throughout the course of Lyme disease treatment, as many treatments cause nausea and vomiting. THC may also be helpful in cases of Mycoplasma Pneumoniae and other infections that inhibit respiratory functioning by acting as a bronchodilator and dilating the bronchi and bronchioles, thereby increasing airflow to the lungs and alleviating resistance in the respiratory airway. Furthermore, THC is a stimulant and may aid in combating fatigue—a problem which many individuals with Lyme disease and other chronic illnesses struggle with on a daily basis. Please note: its actions as a stimulant are most prominent in strains containing high amounts of THC, namely, sativa and sativa dominant strains.

Delta-9-tetrayhydrocannabivarin (THCV)

THCV, one of 9 other compounds in cannabis belonging to the delta-9-tetrahydrocannabinol class of cannabinoids, has significant benefits as an analgesic, euphoriant, and antioxidant. THCV is a potential therapy for Parkinson's disease, as it may delay neurodegeneration and reduce symptoms by activating CB2 receptors and blocking CB1 receptors. The 8 other compounds belonging to the delta-9-tetrahydrocannabinol cannabinoids are delta-9-tetrahydrocannabinolic acid A (THCA-A), delta-9-tetrahydrocannabinolic acid B (THCA-B), delta-9-tetrahydrocannabinolic acid-C4 (THCA-C4), delta-9-tetrahydrocannabinol-C4 (THC-C4), delta-9-tetrahydrocannabivarinic acid (THCVA), delta-9-tetrahydrocannabiorcolic acid (THCA-C1), delta-9-tetrahydrocannabiorcol (THC-C1), and delta-7-cis-iso-tetrahydrocannabivarin.

Cannabidiol (CBD)

Cannabidiol, or CBD, is a non-psychoactive cannabinoid found in cannabis that is considered to have a broader spectrum of medicinal uses than THC. CBD has displayed promising results for the treatment of autoimmune disorders, and is an antiepileptic, anticancer, anxiolytic, antipsychotic, analgesic, anti-inflammatory, antidepressant, antimicrobial, antioxidant, and muscle relaxant. The neuroprotective properties in CBD prevent glutamate toxicity, cellular damage, and ischemic damage from insufficient blood flow to the brain.

CBD may be useful in the treatment of Lyme disease and other neurodegenerative disorders that cause oxidative stress because of its potent antioxidant activity and its ability to prevent glutamate toxicity, prevent cellular damage, and protect the brain from ischemic damage. Oxidative stress is often present in neurodegenerative diseases such as Lyme disease, Alzheimer's disease, autism, and chronic fatigue syndrome. Oxidative stress reduces the brain's antioxidant abilities and causes toxic effects in the brain by producing peroxides and free radicals, thus resulting in the damage of all cellular components of the brain including proteins, lipids, and DNA.

CBD is a 5-HT1A serotonin receptor agonist, a type of serotonin receptor impaired by elevated cortisol levels in those with Lyme disease. Activating 5-HT1A serotonin receptors can relieve anxiety and depression, decrease aggression, decrease impulsivity, improve sex drive, prolong REM sleep, and enhance cognitive functions associated with the prefrontal cortex of the brain. CBD's interaction with 5-HT1A serotonin receptors is responsible for its use as an antidepressant, anxiolytic, and neuroprotectant.

The Role of THC and CBD in Th1/Th2 Conditions

T-helper cells (Th) are lymphocytes, or white blood cells, that recognize foreign pathogens. In the case of autoimmune conditions, they mistakenly recognize normal tissues as foreign pathogens, prompting the body to wage war on itself.

When a foreign pathogen is recognized, T-helper cells respond by producing cytokines, which are hormonal messenger proteins responsible for biological functions in the immune system. T-helper cells are grouped into two categories, characterized by what type of cytokines they produce. Th1 lymphocytes produce type 1 cytokines like interleukin-2 (IL-2), tumor necrosis factor-beta (TNF-b), and interferon-gamma (INF-gama). Th2 lymphocytes produce cytokines like interleukin-4, 5, 6, 10, and 13 (IL-4, IL-5, IL-6, IL-10, IL-13). Typically, the Th1/Th2 ratio in healthy individuals is mostly balanced. In the case of an illness, a stronger response is provoked in one group of t-helper cells than in the other, creating either a Th1 or Th2 dominance.

Lyme disease disrupts the balance of Th1/Th2 upon infection, at which point a strong Th1 response is initiated, classifying it as a Th1 condition. Some fear that cannabis will shift Lyme disease into a Th2 condition, as both CBD and THC shift immune response from Th1 to Th2. However, a shift from Th1 towards Th2 response occurs primarily when cannabis is smoked. Generally speaking, the shift from Th1 to Th2 is not significant and occurs primarily in the lungs. However, in the case of conditions impacting the lungs, such as Lyme disease co-infections like Mycoplasma Pneumoniae and related conditions like mold toxicity, it is important to avoid immunosuppression in the lungs when at all possible, rendering smoking as the least desirable option for cannabis use. It is worth noting that there is evidence that balancing Th1/Th2 complexes in those with chronic Lyme disease improves treatment outcomes. So, slightly provoking a Th2 response with cannabis may actually be of benefit by reducing Th1 dominance to some degree. This is a largely unexamined theory worth exploring.

Cannabinol (CBN)

One of the most fascinating characteristics of CBN, a breakdown product of THC, is its aptness as a formidable analgesic. Its analgesic properties are so strong that its effects are three times as powerful as those of aspirin. Like aspirin, though, it is non psychoactive. CBN also works as a sedative, causing drowsiness and offering relief to those with sleep disorders such as insomnia.

Cannabigerol (CBG)

CBG, the first cannabinoid ever identified, acts as a biogenetic precursor to all other cannabinoids. It induces drowsiness and helps individuals who experience difficulties falling asleep. Large quantities of CBG are found in hashish, a byproduct of cannabis discussed in further detail in the upcoming chapter on forms and methods of cannabis use. CBG is an antimicrobial, making it profitable for treating bacterial and fungal infections. A precursor to CBG called cannabigerolic acid (CBGA) has a prominent pharmacological characteristic as an antibiotic agent.

Cannabichromene (CBC)

CBC enhances the effects of THC. It behaves as a sedative, analgesic, and anti-inflammatory. Considering most cannabinoids with medicinal benefits display analgesic properties, it is clear why cannabis proves to be a useful treatment for pain management for many individuals. The antifungal properties of CBC make it a prominent resource for targeting Candida overgrowth in the body. CBC's ability to function as an antibiotic, similar to various other chemical components found in cannabis, lends to the plant's potent antibacterial qualities. Also, in cases of heavy metal toxicity, please note that the body creates an overgrowth of Candida to absorb the metals as a survival instinct. So, if you use cannabis and have Candida, please be aware the elimination of excess Candida may simultaneously prompt the release of heavy metals. That, paired with the antibacterial and antimicrobial properties of cannabis, makes implementing a thorough detoxification program an essential factor when using cannabis to treat Lyme disease. Do not underestimate the powerful bactericidal and fungicidal effects of cannabis, and the importance of supporting the body with thorough, and if necessary rigorous, detoxification methods.

Terpenes

Terpenes, the primary chemical constituents in essential oils of various plants and flowers, are responsible for the unique aroma of cannabis. Terpenes with naturally altered chemical structures, also known as terpenoids, are key building blocks for cannabinoids. Currently, over 120 different terpenes have been identified in cannabis. The number and variety of terpenes which any given cannabis plant contains is strain specific, with each varying, sometimes greatly, depending on the chemical makeup of the strain. Biologically speaking, terpenes in cannabis display a wide range of medicinal benefits, including, but not limited to, anti-inflammatory, antibiotic, and analgesic properties. Terpenes and terpenoids in cannabis appear to work synergistically with one another. That is, their effects are more powerful when they are utilized collectively rather than as isolated specimens. Among the most medicinally beneficial terpenes in cannabis are myrcene, caryophyllene, limonene, linalool, pulegone, cineole, pinene, and borneol.

Myrcene

Myrcene is the most prevalent terpene in cannabis. Myrcene modulates permeability of cell membranes, enabling more THC to reach the brain cells. It acts as an antimicrobial, antioxidant, antiseptic, anti-carcinogen, anti-inflammatory, anti-depressant, and analgesic. It is a powerful muscle relaxant, making it useful for those with muscle related symptoms like spasticity or spasms. Myrcene also enhances antibiotic properties of other terpenes and terpenoids against certain strains of bacteria, including Staphylococcus aureus, Bacillus subtilis, Pseudomonas aeruginosa, and Escherichia coli.

By acting as an antimutagenic, myrcene inhibits spontaneous mutation of cells, a phenomenon often responsible for the onset of various types of cancer. This is relevant to those with Lyme disease and related conditions, as evidence indicates that people with Lyme disease, Epstein-Barr virus, Chlamydia pneumoniae, and Mycoplasma pneumoniae have an increased risk of developing Lymphoma, a cancer characterized by development of abnormal blood cell tumors followed by rapid division of more abnormal cells.

Caryophyllene

Although weakly, caryophyllene binds to CB2 receptors. It is a calcium and potassium ion channel blocker that helps alleviate pressure exerted by the heart muscles. Equipped with analgesic and anti-inflammatory properties, caryophyllene displays superb results when applied topically to toothaches and on swollen, painful joints. As a cytoprotective for gastric mucosa, caryophyllene scavenges free radicals, stimulates growth and repair of damaged cells, strengthens the gastric mucosal barrier, and enhances blood flow of gastric mucosa. Satureja montana essential oil, which is rich in caryophyllene and another terpene called terpineol, demonstrates moderate antimalarial effects and is a perfect example of how terpenes are often more potent when operating in a synergistic nature.

Limonene

Limonene is a cannabinoid receptor agonist, immune potentiator, antidepressant, and antimutagenic. A puissant antifungal and anticarcinogenic, limonene intervenes as a protective shield against aspergillus fungi and carcinogens produced by smoking cannabis. Therefore, limonene is thought to reduce potential harmful effects from smoking cannabis (**to what degree it does so is strain specific, so do not assume you are entirely protected from any possible harmful effects of smoking cannabis).

Synergistically, limonene works alongside other terpenes, yielding a wide range of biological benefits. By rapidly penetrating cell membranes, limonene encourages cellular absorption of other terpenes, resulting in enhanced systolic blood pressure. Another favorable synergistic effect between limonene and other terpenes is the ability to inhibit the growth of various types of bacteria and fungi.

Limonene was the primary constituent in an essential oil mix implemented in a clinical study conducted by the Department of Psychiatry at Mie University School of Medicine in Japan on the effects of citrus fragrance on immune function and depressive states.[3] Researchers found that, in some depression sufferers, an essential oil rich in limonene significantly reduces the amount of antidepressants needed to manage their depression.

Linalool

Although linalool accounts for less than 5 percent of terpenes in cannabis, it nonetheless exhibits impressively powerful biological functions as a sedative, antidepressant, anxiolytic, and immune potentiator. In conjunction with other terpenes and terpenoids, linalool helps alleviate THC induced anxiety. Of course, like virtually all other medicinal effects and characteristics of cannabis and its chemical constituents, the extent to which it does so is entirely strain dependent, with the specific chemical makeup of each strain serving as the deciding factor. Together, linalool and other terpenes and terpenoids strengthen immune function by inhibiting secretion of hypothalamic-pituitary-adrenal (HPA) stress hormones like corticosterone, essentially resulting in reduced levels of anxiety and depression.

Pulegone

Pulegone promotes the brain's ability to store memories by hindering acetylcholinesterase, an enzyme that destroys acetylcholine, a neurotransmitter that helps the brain store memories. Pulegone is also mucolytic, and helps break up congestion in the respiratory system. It has sedative and antipyretic effects as well.

Cineole

Cineole, which is also found in rosemary and eucalyptus, is a minor constituent in cannabis with major medicinal benefits. Among them are its abilities to relieve pain and inflammation, increase cerebral brain flow, enhance cortical activity, serve as an analgesic, lessen pain sensation by acting as an antinociceptive, and cross the blood brain barrier to quickly activate an olfactory reaction. Cineole displays remarkable antifungal properties against Candida albicans, Cryptococcus neoformans, and Trichophyton mentagrophytes. Its medical benefits do not end there, though. Not only does it also possess antibacterial properties against infections like Bacillus subtilis, Escherichia coli, and Staphylococcus aureus, but a study on rats showed it prevents sexual transmission of Herpes Simplex Virus Type 2 (HSV-2) as well.[4]

Pinene

Pinene has various medicinal qualities. Among the most outstanding is its ability to inhibit and reverse memory loss, thereby aiding those with Alzheimer's disease and other neurodegenerative disorders that cause memory loss. It does so by preventing the occurrence of acetylcholinesterase, an enzyme that destroys acetylcholine (a molecule utilized by the brain for processing and storing information). As a result, pinene aids in both the restoration of lost memories and the retention of new ones. It also enhances cognitive functioning and serves as an impressive expectorant and topical antiseptic.

Borneol

Borneol has calming, sedative effects. It is used medicinally in China to aid in recovery from illness and stress. Easing biological consequences of stress not only significantly increases the odds of healing from an illness, but it decreases the risk of contracting new infections as well. Interestingly, natural borneol plant extracts are used to repel insects—which, as you likely know, transmit infectious diseases like Lyme disease and Lyme disease co-infections.

Flavonoids

At least 23 polyphenolic compounds known as flavonoids have been identified in cannabis. They are equipped with a wide range of health benefits, including antiviral, anti-allergic, anti-inflammatory, antitumor, and antioxidant properties. Flavonoids inhibit oxidative cell damage, prevent blood cells from rupturing, and help strengthen the immune system by enhancing the effects of Vitamin C. Another health benefit of flavonoids is that they block free radicals by chelating iron ions that create them. To do so, they promote fenton reactions, scavenge superoxide anions, and extinguish alkoxy and peroxyl radicals. Indicators your body needs more flavonoids include frequent colds and infections, bruising easily, frequent nosebleeds, and abnormal swelling from injuries. Unlike most flavonoids, which are found in a variety of plants, Cannaflavin A and B are unique to cannabis. Currently, the following flavonoids in cannabis have the most known health benefits:

Apigenin

Apigenin, a flavonoid found in most vascular plants, exhibits a wealth of properties advantageous to biological processes of the human body. Apigenin is a strong anxiolytic, meaning it helps ease symptoms of anxiety. With apigenin as its primary anxiolytic agent, chamomile is an excellent testament to the power of the anxiolytic qualities of apigenin. By binding to central benzodiazepine receptors in the brain, apigenin soothes symptoms of anxiety without causing memory loss, fatigue, sedation, or any of the other host of undesirable side effects accompanying the use of synthetic benzodiazepines like Ativan or Xanax (**please note, lethargic and sedating effects from other compounds in cannabis may overshadow those of apigenin). Apigenin also has anticancer properties and is especially beneficial for treating breast cancer, as it inhibits antiestrogen-resistant breast cancer cell growth.[5] Among the other health benefits of apigenin are its actions as a formidable anti-inflammatory, helping to alleviate numerous uncomfortable and/or dangerous symptoms resulting from inflammation of the brain or body.

Quercetin

The antioxidant properties of quercetin are more powerful than those of any other flavonoid. Its antioxidant effects are amplified when combined with other antioxidants. Quercetin is also an antimutagenic, antineoplastic, and antiviral.

Cannaflavin A and B

Cannaflavin A and B are flavonoids unique to the cannabis plant. Both lessen symptoms of rheumatoid arthritis by preventing rheumatoid synovial cells from producing prostaglandin E2, which are biologically active lipids that aid in progression of rheumatoid arthritis. Cannaflavin A is also known for inhibiting cyclooxygenase enzymes (COX) and lipoxygenase enzymes (LO).

β-sitosterol (Beta Sitosterol)

Possessing a chemical structure similar to cholesterol, β-sitosterol is able to significantly reduce the amount of cholesterol absorbed by the gut. By reducing acute inflammation, β-sitosterol helps ease flares of arthritis symptoms and other inflammatory conditions. It also has properties as a 5 a-reductase inhibitor, and is a valuable tool for treating benign prostatic hyperplasia.

Chapter 3

SPECIES AND STRAINS OF CANNABIS

The plant genus Cannabis has three species, each with different chemical constituents and medicinal properties. Cannabis Sativa and Cannabis Indica are the two most commonly used species. The third species of cannabis, C. Ruderalis, grows wild in Europe and Russia and is rarely used. It has a relatively small stature and contains low amounts of THC (tetrahydrocannabinol), making it of lesser demand. The majority of present day cannabis is derived from the Sativa and Indica species. These two species and the numerous strains they are made up of are the ones of primary focus throughout this book. They are fundamentally different chemically, medicinally, and physiologically.

Hybrids

Accounting for the vast majority of cannabis strains are "hybrids" consisting of a combination of Indica and Sativa. The percentages of Indica and Sativa in any given hybrid vary greatly, with their ratios ultimately depending on the grower's intended use of the strain. For example, when intending to harvest a strain to alleviate a specific medical condition such as insomnia, the desired end result will likely contain a dominant proportion of Indica rather than Sativa, as Indica has sedative effects and Sativa has mentally stimulating ones.

C. Ruderalis

Although C. Ruderalis is rarely used, due to its small size and low THC potency, having general knowledge of its basic characteristics may nonetheless prove useful. Commercial crossbred hybrids consisting of all three species of cannabis are sometimes cultivated in order to create an "autoflowering" plant. Autoflowering, a characteristic specific to the C. Ruderalis species of cannabis, provides growers with a harvesting advantage—the plant is able to progress from vegetative growth to the flowering stage automatically as it ages, unlike season dependent, photoperiodic plants such as Sativa and Indica. Harvesting photoperiodic plants depends on the ratio of light to dark hours in a twenty-four hour period, making their cultivation seasonal. Hybrids with C. Ruderalis, on the other hand, produce numerous harvests in one season alone and can grow in environments that would place photoperiodic plants like Indica and Sativa under too much stress.

Producing hybrids from a combination of all three species of cannabis is ideal for certain medical needs, namely ones requiring high contents of CBD and low contents of THC, as C. Ruderalis only contains approximately 20 percent THC. Still, an estimated 99 percent of hybrids are void of C. Ruderalis and are derived purely from combinations of Indica and Sativa.

Sativa

Effects of Sativa are more cerebral than physical. Sativa produces a stimulating "mental" high, which can enhance creativity, concentration, and focus. The euphoric, uplifting high induced by Sativa makes it, or a hybrid dominant in it, the ideal strain for depression and/or stress.

Cannabis Sativa originated in Southeast Asia. Sativa plants thrive in warmer climates and are tall, thin plants physically distinguishable from Indica plants. They have narrower leaves and are taller than Indica plants, generally maturing between 6 and 12 feet tall. Sativa's cannabinoid profile contains high levels of THC and low levels of CBD. High levels of THC in Sativa are responsible for its stimulating, euphoric effects, as well as its benefits as an anti-epileptic, anti-cancer, anti-emetic, anti-depressant, anti-inflammatory, appetite stimulant, analgesic, and hypotensive agent. Since Sativa tends to have low levels of CBD, which is a potent anti-bacterial, utilizing non-psychoactive CBD oil in combination with Sativa or Sativa dominant strains may maximize antibacterial effects.

Indica

Cannabis Indica produces more of a "body" high than Sativa, with effects that are more physical than cerebral. This makes it an ideal strain for pain relief, sedation, and relaxation. While Sativa can be helpful for those suffering from depression, Indica is more ideal for those suffering from anxiety due to its sedative properties. The "laid-back" drowsy feeling it induces can increase laziness and decrease productivity, potentially worsening symptoms of depression.

Indica is believed to have originated in the Middle East in Pakistan and Afghanistan, primarily in the Hindu Kush Mountain Range. Indica plants, which thrive in cooler climates than Sativa, are physically distinguishable from Sativa plants. They are usually a darker shade of green, have broader leaves, and are shorter—reaching around 3 to 5 feet high on average. Indica's chemical profile is more balanced than that of Sativa, consisting of higher amounts of CBD. This makes Indica dominant strains more ideal than Sativa ones for use as a pain reliever, sleep aid, and muscle relaxant.

Chapter 4

FORMS AND METHODS OF USE

IMPORTANT NOTE TO THE READER: This chapter contains forms and methods of use which have not been validated by clinical trials or safety studies. Much of the information in this chapter is experimental and anecdotal. Use of this information is at your own risk. Do not purchase or use cannabis products unless they are legal in your region. It is strongly recommended that the information in this chapter only be used under the close supervision of a licensed physician.

Various forms and methods of cannabis are utilized for consumption, each varying in effects depending on the individual, sometimes significantly. When the bud of the plant is consumed in raw form, it is typically smoked with a pipe or, on the healthier end of the spectrum, inhaled as vapor from a vaporizer. However, cannabis is often made into other forms including, but not limited to, oils, edibles, waxes, juices, teas, salves, and lotions. Some forms are consumed internally, while others are applied externally as topicals. Which method of use is "best" is almost entirely a matter of personal preference. Our bodies are all unique and respond differently to different methods of treatment. The method of use I find most beneficial may be of lesser benefit to someone else, and vice versa. For example, I find the effects of edibles and cannabis infused coconut or olive oil to be the most favorable of all methods of consumption, and smoking to be the least. On the other hand, I have heard various accounts from people claiming they had horrible, anxiety laden experiences with edibles, usually as a result of consuming too much due to the delayed onset of edibles from digestion, which will be covered in further depth within this chapter. Also, I am not a medical doctor, so I do not advise people on which method is best.

Smoking

While the almost instantaneous effects of smoking cannabis are certainly an upside when in need of fast relief from uncomfortable symptoms, the long term consequences of doing so certainly qualify as a downside. Although smoking cannabis on a regular basis may potentially damage the lungs (an issue which there is some debate over), it is still not nearly as harmful as smoking cigarettes. Placing the two in the same category, as those who protest legalization of cannabis do, is far from fair or logical. If the legal substance, tobacco, is killing people and damaging their health, while the illegal one has actually proven to save lives, then current laws and a large portion of society's reasoning abilities are very much skewed. The September 2003 issue of The British Medical Journal references two large studies proving cannabis smoke does not kill people, concluding there is no such thing as fatal overdose from cannabis.[1] The journal does point out that a

2001 study suggests there is an increased risk of heart attack for up to one hour after smoking cannabis. However, this seems to be extremely rare, accounting for less than one-fifth of 1 percent of heart attacks.

Vaporizing

"Vaping" is considered a healthy alternative to smoking cannabis. Inhaling cannabis from a vaporizer—as opposed to from a pipe, bong, or joint, also known as a "cannabis cigarette"—exposes you to a considerably less amount of harmful toxins. By slowly heating the herb, vaporizers release as many active ingredients of cannabis as smoking does, but with fewer harmful byproducts. When smoking, the herb is burned at a high temperature and heated rapidly, causing the plant material to combust, paving the way for release of harmful toxins and carcinogens. Since vaporizers heat cannabis in a more gentle manner, the plant material is not combusted as it is when smoking, enabling active ingredients of the cannabis plant to be emitted through a stream of vapor void of the amount of harmful byproducts potentially inhaled when smoking. Furthermore, you get up to 95 percent of the cannabinoids in the product you are consuming when you vape it, compared to a measly 10 percent when you smoke it.

Hemp, or Hempseed, Oil

There is a lot of confusion over the differences between "hemp," "marijuana," and "cannabis." Hemp is a non-psychoactive product derived from the stalk and seeds of the cannabis plant, while what is considered actual "marijuana" (or "cannabis") is derived from the dried leaves and flowers of the plant. To be clear, both are from the cannabis plant. Aside from the parts of the plant used to make them, other major differences between hemp and marijuana are their chemical properties and intended uses. When referring to oils, many confuse hemp oil with hash oil, but there are distinct differences between the two, ranging from production, benefits, chemical composition, and methods of use. While hemp oil is made with seeds from cannabis, hash oil is made from the cannabis flower. Trace amounts of THC have been detected in some samples of hemp oil, but not enough to induce psychoactive effects. However, it has a high concentration of CBD, making it a more enticing option than other cannabis products for those who wish to avoid the psychoactive effects of other cannabis products.

Hemp oil is produced by pressing seeds of the cannabis plant and using pressure to release the oil. Although Sativa used to be the standard species of cannabis used for producing hemp oil, hemp oils are now being made from Indica seeds as well. Two kinds of hemp oil exist: unrefined and refined. Ranging from dark to light green in color, unrefined oil has a nutty flavor with a grassy undertone. The darker the oil is, the grassier the flavor tends to be. Refined hemp oil is clear, has little to no flavor and no natural vitamins or antioxidants. Refined hemp oil is found in lotions, face wash, soaps, shampoos, conditioners and other body products. Industrially, it is found in lubricant, paint, ink, fuel, and plastic products. Numerous organizations also promote the use of hemp oil for mass production of biodiesel.

Hemp oil is rich in essential fatty acids (EFAs) linoleic acid (LA), a polyunsaturated omega-6 fatty acid, and alpha-linolenic acid (ALA), a polyunsaturated omega-3 acid. Although the EFAs gamma-linolenic acid, an omega-6 fatty acid, and stearidonic acid, an omega-3 fatty acid, are also present in hemp oil, they are far less abundant than LA and ALA. With the same 3:1 balanced ratio of omega-3 to omega-6 EFAs required by the human body for maximum health, taking 1 tablespoon of hemp oil a day provides the body with the proper balance of omega-6 (LA) and omega-3 (ALA) EFAs needed to maintain optimal bodily functioning. Its ability to do so is superior to that of flaxseed oil, as it can be used on a regular basis without resulting in a deficiency or imbalance of EFAs in the body.

**Hemp oil comes in both liquid and capsule forms. You can also find hemp based lotions, shampoos, salves, and other body products. They should be legal, but always double check.

Hash

Hash is a staple in the world of cannabis. It is far more potent than other forms of cannabis, as it contains concentrated amounts of the psychoactive ingredient THC, as well as many other cannabinoids, depending on the hash. Of course, the exact percentage of THC varies significantly among products, depending on the unique composition of essential oils, terpenes, cannabinoids, and actual THC content in the specific strain used to produce the oil. There are also variants of traditional hash oil, such as the popular hash derived products known as butane hash oil (BHO), bubble hash, wax, and shatter.

To produce traditional hash, resin glands are shaken off cannabis flowers or "buds" onto silver screens to create kief, which has a significantly higher concentration of psychoactive cannabinoids, like THC, than the cannabis flowers it is derived from. Normally, the kief is then compressed, forming a block of hash. However, both kief and compressed forms of hash are available for purchase in states where cannabis is legal. The most notable difference between the two is that one is compressed into a hard block, while the other one, kief, has a loose powder-like consistency.

Butane Hash Oil (BHO)

To make butane hash oil, an immensely potent hash concentrate, a solvent is used to extract resin from cannabis buds. Using a tube filled with cannabis plant matter, liquid butane is passed through, picking up crystal resins along the way. Then, the butane and resin crystals acquired, or the "solvent," exit the tube into a glass jar. Since butane is a volatile molecule that boils at -1°C, only crystallized resins are left in the jar after the solvent is boiled. To purge any possible butane still trapped in the oil, the crystallized resins are collected from the jar and are then vacuum purged in a vacuum chamber. Depending on the purging process (i.e. length of time in vacuum chamber and the amount of heat used), butane hash oil is made into different forms characterized by texture, such as oil, wax, crumble, shatter, dab, or budder.

Solvents other than butane that are commonly used include dry ice CO_2, ethanol, isopropyl alcohol, and hexane. Medically speaking, ethanol and dry ice CO_2 oils are the healthiest solvents for making hash oil. Solvents like butane can leave remains of heavy metals behind in the finished product. Please read through the next section on CO_2 oil for a more in depth explanation as to why this is so.

CO2 Oil

Beneficial essences from cannabis plant material are commonly extracted with CO_2 (carbon dioxide) to form cannabis concentrates. The method used to make CO_2 oil, a variant of hash oil, is the same method used for producing pure essential oils and for stripping out and isolating single botanical oils. While I covered hash oil made with butane as a solvent earlier, and listed other options for solvents, I think it is of the utmost importance to reiterate that CO_2 is probably a much safer and healthier solvent to use than butane and other solvents, at least when it comes to using hash for medical purposes. *Once again, CO_2 tends to be a much safer solvent than butane when making oil, with ethanol following close behind.* Due to its place in nature, CO_2 is a natural solvent that leaves behind no harmful byproducts or residues. Butane, on the other hand, can potentially leave heavy metals in the finished product.

For CO_2 extraction, also referred to as "Super Fluid Extraction" or "SFE," high pressure is used to force carbon dioxide through the plant matter. Pushing carbon dioxide through plant matter at a high pressure makes precise separation of plant matter possible, allowing for isolation of the purest essence of cannabis. The resulting oil is transparent with an amber tint to it.

Cannabis Infused Coconut or Olive Oil

Cannabis infused coconut and olive oils are abundant in benefits, especially for those with Lyme disease and associated conditions—so much so that it was a combination of both cannabis infused coconut oil and cannabis infused olive oil that pushed me over my last "hump" in the process of healing from Lyme disease, shifting me into remission within a matter of months. However, after becoming symptom free, I discontinued use entirely. For me, this proved to be a mistake, allowing for the reemergence of symptoms. I now feel it is crucial to stay on a maintenance dose of oil, indefinitely.

The process of making cannabis infused coconut or olive oil is incredibly simple, embarrassingly so really, even for someone like myself who is among the world's worst cooks. The recipe for making cannabis infused coconut or olive oil is, like I said, incredibly simple and is, what I deem, a safe process that can be done from the ease of one's own kitchen in as little as 20 minutes.

Many have asked me for the recipe for making cannabis infused coconut or olive oil. So, I have listed the specific steps I used to make it below *for those who live in locations where cannabis use is legal.* The ingredient amounts listed are sufficient for making a small batch, although it lasted me around a month. In order to make a smaller or larger batch, just adjust the ratios accordingly:

- Using either a grinder designed specifically for cannabis, or even a simple coffee grinder, grind 2 tablespoons of dried cannabis buds (leaves and flowers) of your strain of choice until the herb is finely powdered.

- Next, mix the powdered herb with ¾ cups of coconut or olive oil. Place the mixture in a pot on the stove to simmer for approximately 20 minutes, and stir it frequently. *Please note: simmer means to heat something until it is almost boiling, but not actually boiling, and to then keep it at that temperature. The oil should never be boiled, only simmered.*

- After simmering for 20 minutes, turn off the stove and allow the oil to sit and cool for approximately 30 minutes.

- Once the oil is cooled, strain and filter the oil into a bottle or jar using a strainer such as a coffee filter—an empty herbal tincture bottle works fantastically for storage purposes, allowing for ease in consumption and dosage management with a dropper, as well as for ease in traveling with it in a purse or bag.

When implementing cannabis infused coconut or olive oil into your daily health routine, it is highly recommended that you do so gradually, initially taking the minimum possible amount and slowly increasing the dose over time, similar to taking any other herb. For example, in the case of taking it out of an herbal tincture bottle with a dropper, the starting dose would literally be one drop. For some people, the body will react fairly quickly, so if there are no noticeable and/or adverse reactions within thirty minutes to an hour of taking the first drop, another can be added. Other people may have more delayed reactions, so proceed with caution and only under the care of your physician. This process is repeated until the appropriate dose is found, which differs for everyone. The body is really the only guideline for dosing (I believe this to be true for most things), and will make it clear what it does and does not want if listened to.

Many ask if it is more beneficial to use cannabis infused coconut oil or olive oil to treat Lyme disease and Lyme disease co-infections. My answer is this: I feel both are wonderfully healing, each with their own properties specific to problems faced by those with Lyme disease, Lyme co-infections, and related conditions. Coconut oil, for example, is an all-around great medicine as it kills bacteria, viruses, and fungi. That it kills fungi is, of course, very beneficial for those with Candida albicans—which, in regards to those with Lyme disease and Lyme disease co-infections, is most people. Coconut oil is also a good source of vitamin b6. People with the biochemical disorder Pyroluria (also known as HPU/KPU), a condition which an estimated 80 percent of people with chronic and persistent Lyme disease have, are severely deficient in b6, rendering cannabis infused coconut oil an advantageous option for those who have this condition—*Please note, some with pyroluria require a specific form of b6 called P5P (Pyridoxal-5-Phosphate). So, this does not apply to those people.* When it comes to cannabis infused olive oil, those with Mycoplasma are in luck. Mycoplasma scavenges nutrients, and olive oil helps reverse the resulting malnutrition. So, not only are the numerous benefits of cannabis itself reaped, ones from olive oil are as well.

In the case of Lyme disease and Lyme co-infections, both cannabis infused coconut and olive oils are immensely beneficial. Since they are simple to make, making small batches of both and then testing to see which the body responds best to is a practical way to determine which oil is best because, as we know, no two cases of Lyme disease and Lyme co-infections are identical in nature.

Cannabis Tonics and Tinctures

Cannabis tonics and tinctures are made by soaking the flowered tops and leaves of cannabis in an alcohol solution, essentially transferring THC and other cannabinoids into the liquid solution. Any solid particles of plant matter left in the solution are then drained out. Tinctures and tonics are added to food, consumed orally by placing drops of it directly under the tongue, or applied to the skin (i.e. in the case of painful, swollen joints, an individual may choose to rub the tincture or tonic directly on their knees as a topical pain reliever). When suffering from nausea and vomiting, tinctures and tonics are a great option for cannabis use, due to their various means of application and consumption.

Edibles

Cannabis edibles are made with cannabis infused oil or butter, also known as "cannabutter." To make cannabis infused oils to cook edibles with, simmer flowered tops and leaves of the cannabis plant in coconut or olive oil for approximately 20 minutes (in depth recipe and instructions listed in the previous section titled "Cannabis Infused Coconut or Olive Oil") To make cannabutter to cook edibles with, simmer the flowered tops and leaves of cannabis in butter for several hours. These processes transfer THC and other cannabinoids into the butter or oil. The resulting butter or oil is then used to cook a wide variety of foods ranging from brownies, cookies, candies, muffins, and liquids such as soup.

Keep in mind that the effects of edibles differ from those of other forms of cannabis use, such as vaporizing or smoking. The effects take longer to kick in, which can result in over-consumption from thinking that you have not eaten enough and need to eat more because you do not immediately feel the effects. To be safe, wait at least an hour before eating more. Just as the effects of edibles take longer to kick in, they also take longer to wear off. While edibles are excellent for various health problems, such as pain, insomnia, and muscle stiffness and spasticity, they are clearly not ideal when seeking relief from nausea or vomiting.

Cannabis Tea

The process of preparing cannabis tea is similar to that of other herbal teas. Boiling water is poured into a pot containing plant material (cannabis stems, leaves, and/or buds). However, unlike traditional herbal teas, an extra step unique to cannabis tea is required for preparation. Since THC is only mildly soluble in water, a solvent like alcohol, butter, or oil must be added in order to extract THC from the plant matter. The tea must steep for at least 30 minutes. Cannabis teas are psychoactive and vary in strength, depending on the ratio of cannabis to water that is used. The ideal potency depends on personal preference and tolerability. Depending on the potency of the tea, effects range from mild, inducing a slightly sedative effect similar in nature to valerian root tea, to strong, inducing an extremely sedating effect that lasts for hours.

CBD Oil

A relatively new line of cannabis products made from the stalk and seeds of the cannabis plant, called CBD oil, are an option for those who live in states where cannabis use is illegal, as CBD oil does not contain the psychoactive ingredient THC—if it does, it only contains trace amounts, which are not enough to cause an alteration in mental status. Still, for this reason, you may wish to double check products before purchasing them. Since CBD oil consists only of the cannabinoid Cannabidiol (CBD) and is void of psychoactive ingredients like THC (unless it has trace amounts, as discussed above) and other cannabinoids, terpenes, flavonoids and so on, it possesses less benefits than actual marijuana. However, since CBD oil itself does have some benefits, it is certainly a great option for those who cannot legally obtain cannabis but still wish to gain some of the medicinal benefits of the plant. Additionally, products consisting of CBD extracts can be found in forms other than oil, such as salves, which I personally find effective for topical pain relief.

Chapter 5

SAFETY OF CANNABIS USE

IMPORTANT NOTE TO THE READER: Please do not use cannabis products without first conducting additional safety research, and without first consulting your physician. Use of this information is at your own risk. The information in this chapter (and book) are not intended to serve as medical advice nor is it intended to replace the care of a licensed physician. This chapter is not exhaustive in its treatment of cannabis safety; there are other important considerations not included herein.

The safety of cannabis use is a topic of great debate, with those opposed to it claiming it is a gateway drug, harmful to the brain, and more. There is some truth to these claims, which we will cover herein. Other concerns include overdose, toxicity, acute effects, allergies, interactions with other drugs, bacteria, pesticides, mold exposure, and legal factors, to name a few. Surely, there are other concerns as well. However, the aforementioned are among the most prominent ones and are worth further examination.

Overdose/Toxicity

The possibility of overdose or toxicity from cannabis is often a major concern of those opposed to its legalization, as well as those considering using it themselves for medicinal purposes, and rightfully so. Americans For Safe Access, a group dedicated to educating the public on various aspects of cannabis use, state that for a person to overdose on cannabis, they would have to smoke approximately 1,500 pounds in 15 minutes.[1] Rest assured, this has been ruled physically impossible.

Gateway Drug

That cannabis use is a gateway to abusing harder drugs is also an understandable concern, but the validity behind it is questionable. Almost any substance can be seen as a "gateway drug." For example, soda, energy drinks, coffee, and caffeinated products in general have been labeled by some as gateway drugs for cocaine and methamphetamine use. The same could be said of alcohol. In my opinion, the problem is not so much the substance itself as much as it is an individual's personality or predisposition for addiction.

Some people have addictive personalities. If all things that supposedly serve as gateway drugs or have potential to be addictive were made illegal, we would live in a very limited world—more so than we already do—and our economy would crash—more so than it already has. Sugar, caffeine, processed food, tobacco products, and a large majority of both pharmaceutical and over the counter drugs would be illegal. That they are not begs me to ask the question: is the concern that cannabis is a gateway drug a real one for all who voice it, or is it a mere scapegoat masking deeper ulterior motivations for some? The answer to this will likely remain unclear and up for speculation indefinitely. Really, all we need to focus on is using logic and reasoning to the best of our abilities in all we do, including in the use of cannabis to treat medical conditions.

Acute Side Effects of Cannabis Use

If inhaled, onset of acute effects of cannabis are almost immediate. With other methods of consumption, such as edibles, effects may take up to an hour to set in. Acute effects include dry mouth, red eyes, blurred vision, delayed motor skills, sedation, and anxiety. Anxiety and panic attacks have been of great concern for many with Lyme disease who have considered treating with cannabis. Cannabis can absolutely cause anxiety attacks so intense you become certain of your impending death, as THC directly affects the fear center of your brain, the amygdala. The brains of many with Lyme disease are stuck in a constant fight or flight mode, which cannabis may amplify. The extent to which it does so is highly dependent on the chemical makeup of the strain used, as well as the method of consumption, and the individual biochemistry of the user.

Personally, I have experienced acute, extreme anxiety when using Sativa dominant strains. This is not at all strange or uncommon considering Sativa is THC dominant. Other methods of use, like oils or edibles, and other strains, specifically Indica dominant ones, do not cause me to feel anxious. After meditating on a regular basis, though, I found myself able to tolerate treatment with Sativa dominant strains by meditating until the effects wore off.

Some literature refers to a phenomenon called "marijuana psychosis," in which a person experiences acute episodes of psychosis after marijuana use. This is why it is so crucial to take it slow when increasing intake, starting with the lowest dose possible, and testing out different strains to find which ones works best for you. It is unwise to assume that what works well for another person will work equally as well for you.

**Note: Cannabis can increase heart rate for up to an hour after consumption. Therefore, those with heart problems should proceed with caution, and should only do so after consulting with a medical professional.

Allergies

Avoid using cannabis if you are sensitive or allergic to cannabinoids or plants in the Cannabaceae family. Though it is not particularly common, asthma, pink eye, and a runny or stuffy nose have occurred in cannabinoid sensitive individuals.

Interactions with Other Drugs, Supplements, and Herbs

- **Medications that affect bleeding**: Cannabis may increase the risk of bleeding when taken with drugs, herbs, or supplements that increase the risk of bleeding. Examples of pharmaceuticals and over the counter drugs that may interact with cannabis and increase the risk of bleeding include aspirin, blood thinners like warfarin or heparin, antiplatelet drugs, and nonsteroidal anti-inflammatory drugs including Ibuprofen, Motrin, Advil, and Aleve. Examples of herbs and supplements that may interact with cannabis and increase the risk of bleeding include garlic, saw palmetto, and Ginkgo Biloba.

- **Blood sugar drugs, herbs, and supplements:** Cannabis may affect blood sugar levels. Use with caution if taking medications that affect blood sugar levels. You should be monitored closely if using cannabis while taking drugs for diabetes, or any herbs or supplements that may affect blood sugar levels.

- **Medications that induce drowsiness**: Cannabis may cause drowsiness and amplify sedative effects of other drugs, herbs, or supplements that cause drowsiness. Examples of such substances include benzodiazepines, barbiturates, narcotics, Valerian root, and Pasque flower.

- **Other possible interactions:** Other drugs cannabis may also interact with include anabolic steroids, anticancer herbs and supplements, antioxidants, anti-epileptic herbs and supplements, central nervous system depressants, corticosteroids, dopamine antagonists, and more.

Interaction considerations: Considering the interactions listed above and the possibility of others, using cannabis with caution and under medical supervision is strongly advised, as is starting with minimal doses to see how your body responds.

Pesticides, Bacteria, and Mold

Cannabis contaminated with bacteria, mold, and/or pesticides is primarily a risk for those who smoke the herb. However, obtaining cannabis from a trusted source is strongly recommended. In the case of Lyme disease, or any condition affecting the immune system, refraining from smoking cannabis and instead using other methods of consumption seems to be one of the most important cautionary steps one can take. Other forms of cannabis like oils and edibles are generally safer options, as harmful byproducts are likely to be boiled off during their preparation.

Pregnancy

Melanie Dreher, the dean of nursing at Rush Medical Center of Chicago, studied the effects of prenatal cannabis exposure on neonates in Jamaica.[2] She followed a group of women who smoked cannabis throughout their pregnancies, along with ones who didn't, and compared neurobehavioral skills of infants from both groups to assess neurobehavioral effects of prenatal exposure to cannabis. Approximately one month after birth, the infants with prenatal exposure to cannabis displayed greater physiological stability than those without exposure. After a year, the most significant difference between the two groups was that the neonates who were prenatally exposed to cannabis exhibited stronger social skills (i.e. had better eye contact and were easier to engage with) than those without prenatal exposure to cannabis. Interestingly, infants whose mothers used cannabis the most heavily while pregnant had the best overall scores on autonomic stability, quality of alertness, irritability, and self-regulation.

Use in Adolescents

The popular idea that cannabis use in adolescents causes brain atrophy, or shrinking of the brain, may be little more than a fallacy. Diffusion tensor imaging (a type of MRI that uses the diffusion of water to more precisely delineate white matter of the brain) indicates that teens who use cannabis do not display any consistent evidence indicating brain damage or hindrances in neurological development due to cannabis. Researchers from The Nathan S. Kline Institute for Psychiatric Research and The Department of Psychiatry at New York University School of Medicine compared brain scans of nine males and one female who regularly use cannabis to ones of nine males and one female who do not use cannabis to determine if cannabis use in adolescents causes brain atrophy.[3] Using measures of whole brain volumes, lateral ventricular volumes, and gray matter volumes of the amygdala-hippocampal complex, superior temporal gyrus, and all temporal lobes, researchers examined the brain scans of both groups for signs of cerebral atrophy or compromised white matter integrity. No evidence of cerebral atrophy or decline in white matter integrity was identified in scans of either group, exposing a belief shattering revelation that shocked many—the notion that cannabis use in adolescents shrinks the brain may be an unfounded hypothesis, and nothing more.

Chapter 6

LEGALITIES OF CANNABIS USE IN THE UNITED STATES

"In 2009, marijuana and its colorful culture came into the mainstream more prominently than at any other time in history, but the old perceptions of those who use it—whether for cancer or before a Phish concert—linger in the minds of politicians, bankers, cops, and every other nonsmoker being asked to accept this formerly underground lifestyle now that it's taken up residence in the storefront next to the local Starbucks."

–Greg Campbell
Pot, Inc.: Inside Medical Marijuana,
America's Most Outlaw Industry.

IMPORTANT NOTE TO THE READER: Please do not rely solely on this information to ascertain whether cannabis is legal in your region. Please be sure that cannabis is legal in your region before purchasing or using it.

As I write this, the war on cannabis rages on. For every person who supports the legalization of cannabis there is someone else who opposes it. The majority of individuals in opposition to legalizing cannabis for medicinal and/or recreational use are from older generations, with younger generations (i.e. those in their teens, twenties, and thirties) accounting for the majority who support legalization. Of course, this is not to say there are not any individuals from older generations who support legalization of cannabis, or from younger generations who are opposed to it. After all, programs like D.A.R.E. repeatedly drilled it into our heads as children that cannabis is bad, conditioning us to believe so.

Currently, cannabis is legal for medicinal use in 23 states, and for both medicinal and recreational use in three states. States where cannabis is legal for medicinal use include Alaska, Arizona, California, Colorado, Connecticut, D.C., Delaware, Hawaii, Illinois, Maine, Maryland, Massachusetts, Michigan, Minnesota, Montana, Nevada, New Hampshire, New Jersey, New Mexico, New York, Oregon, Rhode Island, Vermont, and Washington. To obtain cannabis for medicinal use in these states, you must get a prescription from your doctor and get a medical marijuana card. Your healthcare professional can advise you on how to go about doing so. Cannabis is legal for both medicinal and recreational use in Alaska, Colorado, and Washington, meaning you do not need a prescription to obtain it. You can buy it at dispensaries for recreational use. However, medicinal grade cannabis is more potent than the strains you will find in these dispensaries. Also, the amount which you may legally purchase and have on you at once is typically less in regards to recreational use than it is in regards to medicinal use. If you live in one of these states, be sure to stay up to date on the most current laws regarding cannabis use.

If you live in a state where cannabis is illegal for use of any kind, you may still reap certain benefits of cannabis by using legal cannabis products that do not contain the psychoactive ingredient THC, such as CBD oils, CBD salves, and hemp oil. Currently, cannabis is illegal in Alabama, Arkansas, Florida, Georgia, Idaho, Indiana, Iowa, Kansas, Kentucky, Louisiana, Mississippi, Missouri, Nebraska, North Carolina, North Dakota, Ohio, Oklahoma, Pennsylvania, South Carolina, South Dakota, Tennessee, Texas, Utah, Virginia, West Virginia, Wisconsin, and Wyoming. As of now, legislation for the legalization of cannabis is pending in Florida, North Carolina, Ohio, and Pennsylvania.

PART TWO:

USING CANNABIS TO REDUCE THE SYMPTOMS OF LYME DISEASE AND RELATED CONDITIONS

Chapter 7

JOINT PAIN

Sugarcoating any aspect pertaining to what it is like to live in chronic pain from Lyme disease, Lyme co-infections, or any other chronic illness is not an option. Perhaps this is because every bone in my body has endured excruciating physical pain. This is in no way an attempt to complain. Rather, it is an attempt to be entirely honest and hopefully, in doing so, let you know you are far from alone. There are many forms of pain brought on by Lyme disease, Lyme co-infections and related conditions, including arthritis pain, neuropathy, Fibromyalgia or Fibromyalgia-like pain, crushing migraines, muscle pain, and so on; all of which are nothing short of physically, mentally, and spiritually taxing. This, of course, takes the effects of pain caused by these illnesses to a whole other level. Physical pain that is chronic in nature wears on you over time, making not only your body fatigued, but your brain and spirit as well. When this happens, it is only natural for even the strongest of wills and spirits to become depleted at one point or another.

When an individual undergoes acute, intense physical pain, their adrenaline often spikes, sending their body into fight or flight mode, essentially skyrocketing their cortisol levels. It only makes sense that if acute excruciating pain sends people's bodies into fight or flight mode for a short amount of time, then equally if not more intense pain endured on a long term basis sends the body into a duration of fight or flight mode just as chronic as the pain itself. Constant spikes in adrenaline and cortisol levels correlates strongly with constant states of panic, shock, fear, anxiousness, or aggression—pick your poison. Often, treating the underlying cause of increased adrenaline and cortisol levels, such as pain in this case, simultaneously resolves these psychological issues as well. Personal experience and statistics prove chronic pain relief from any form of pain "management" is short lived, and never managed very well in the first place, if strong discipline and dedication are not used. For me, the only antidote for joint pain from Lyme disease and the unimaginable burning pain from Bartonella was cannabis oil, meditation, and hypnotherapy.

Arthritis and Arthritic like Disorders and Symptoms

Arthritis, or severe joint pain, that migrates and comes and goes for some and is steadily present for others is a prevalent, often debilitating symptom of Lyme disease and related conditions, especially Lyme disease co-infections like Bartonella. In the case of Lyme disease, this is referred to as "Lyme arthritis," and is present in at least 80 percent of chronic Lyme disease patients I speak with. While cannabis can act as an anti-microbial, it can also act as an invitation to pain relief from arthritis related symptoms as you embark on your journey to healing. Cannabis may ease the dark nights polluted with joint pain—the kind of pain that makes it challenging to get deep and restful sleep, or in the worst cases, any sleep at all.

Rheumatologists are increasingly acknowledging the dire need for new, effective methods of pain management for arthritic pain, as current drugs on the market are failing to provide sufficient pain relief for those in severe and debilitating pain. The demand is so great that the first session ever held on the topic, titled "Medical Marijuana and the Rheumatologist," was conducted in 2013 during the annual ACR/ARHP (American College of Rheumatology/Association of Rheumatology Health Professionals) meeting in San Diego. One of the expert speakers on the topic was Jason Mcdougall, PhD, an Associate Professor of Pharmacology and Anesthesia at Dalhousie University in Halifax, Nova Scotia in Canada.[1]

Dr. Mcdougall did not hesitate to firmly state the following un-fortunate yet profound truth, "there is a social stigma attached to cannabis that is not wholly justified. These are serious drugs and we need to take them seriously as a way of managing pain effectively." Mcdougall, who has conducted research on treating the painful symptoms of osteoarthritis with cannabinoids, went on to say, "these endocannabinoids are serious contenders to try and alleviate pain and inflammation in rheumatic diseases. We need to stop sniggering about it and talk about it, and embrace them with the necessary caution of course." [1]

To exercise this necessary caution, an understanding of endocan-nabinoids and their biological functions must first be obtained. This understanding has the potential to unlock the door to ef-fective relief from arthritic pain. The endocannabinoid system is a group of neuromodulator lipids and their receptors located throughout the body. Endocannabinoids are active participants in important physiological processes such as pain interpretation, memory, mood, drug addiction, reward systems in the brain, and metabolic processes, including balance of energy, glucose metab-olism, appetite control, and lipolysis. Perhaps most importantly, endocannabinoids are the system in the body responsible for intercepting the physiological and psychoactive effects of cannabis. Endocannabinoids CB1 (cannabis receptor type 1) and CB2 (cannabis receptor type 2) are of primary importance when considering biological mechanisms in the relationship between endocannabinoids and cannabinoids in the human body; and the role this relationship plays in manifesting a large majority of the medicinal benefits of cannabis, including, in this case, relief from joint pain.

According to a study conducted by researchers from the *University of Nottingham UK*, alongside researchers from the *University of Pittsburgh and Virginia Commonwealth University* in the US, a specific cannabinoid receptor known as the cannabinoid 2 (CB2) receptor is weakened during osteoarthritis, resulting in heightened pain and accelerated progression of the condition. By activating CB2 receptors, cannabinoids help reduce pain from osteoarthritis and slow the rate at which the condition progresses.[2]

Studies on human spines of deceased individuals who had osteoarthritis of the knee revealed they had lower numbers of CB2 receptors. The more progressed the disease was, the lower the levels of CB2 receptors were. In response, *Research UK* and the *National Institutes of Health* funded a study in which researchers activated CB2 receptors in lab rats with osteoarthritis in an attempt to reduce pain. Diseased rats were injected with JWH-133, a non-psychoactive synthetic cannabinoid that binds with and activates CB2 receptors, and the results were nothing short of fascinating.[2]

By increasing CB2 receptors with JWH-133 injections, researchers reduced levels of chemicals responsible for causing inflammation in osteoarthritis, and lowered activity of excitatory nerves in the spine that are stimulated by inflammation. The injections also increased the overall amount of CB2 receptor "message" (MRNA) and protein in nerve cells of the spine. To put it simply, activating cannabinoid receptors drastically reduced inflammation in osteoarthritis, thus reducing pain and increasing the quality of life in afflicted individuals. Furthermore, since patients with late stage osteoarthritis have drastically reduced levels of CB2 receptor "message" in the spine, increasing levels of the CB2 receptor "message" might greatly reduce the severity and rate of progression of the disease.[2]

I sincerely trust you are not a rat, though, and the JWH-133 vaccine is not yet on the market. So, where does this leave you? Equipped with the knowledge that by interacting with the CB1 and CB2 receptors in your body's endocannabinoid system, cannabinoids significantly relieve pain from arthritis and arthritis like conditions, as well as potentially inhibit progression of such conditions. Cannabis Sativa and Sativa dominant strains have a cannabinoid profile consisting of high THC levels and low, if any, CBD levels, making Cannabis Indica or Indica-dominant strains ideal candidates for relieving pain from arthritis. With a more balanced chemical makeup, consisting of moderate levels of THC, CBD, and other cannabinoids, Indica produces a pain relieving body effect. The mental high sparked by Sativa is not likely to provide pain relief at a strength remotely equivalent to that of Indica.

Chapter 8

NERVE PAIN

Nerve pain is a common symptom of Lyme disease and associated conditions, such as Fibromyalgia, which is considered a condition as opposed to a disease because it has no known root cause. Individuals with Lyme disease are constantly misdiagnosed with Fibromyalgia, with practitioners completely failing to dig deeper and find the underlying cause of their ailments. For those diagnosed with Fibromyalgia who are unaware they have Lyme disease, this is, of course, devastating. Originally, Fibromyalgia was characterized by severe, debilitating nerve pain. However, over the past three years, the list of symptoms physicians use to make clinical diagnoses of Fibromyalgia has grown significantly, now including symptoms such as brain fog, chronic fatigue, depression, and muscle stiffness, to name a few. Legit evidence as to what exactly causes Fibromyalgia continues to flat line, while spikes in the number of symptoms and cases of Fibromyalgia with no known root causes continue to surge. Nerve pain is the symptom of Fibromyalgia we will focus on in this chapter. Not surprisingly, individuals with chronic Lyme disease also experience a type of nerve pain (not to mention most other symptoms of Fibromyalgia) similar in nature to that experienced by individuals with Fibromyalgia. Perhaps this is a mere coincidence. Perhaps it is not.

There is one unmistakably distinguishable difference between the overlapping symptoms of Fibromyalgia and Lyme disease, though. The latter has an identified root cause for its existence. So, the following information from studies on the effects of cannabis on nerve pain from Fibromyalgia are riddled with mindfulness that Fibromyalgia often proves to be no more than a term for a set of symptoms for those who have Lyme disease. This is not to say all cases of Fibromyalgia are indeed Lyme disease. Rather, it is simply to say many with Lyme disease are misdiagnosed with Fibromyalgia because the manifestations of their symptoms are close to identical in nature to those required for a clinical diagnosis of Fibromyalgia.

Research on the endocannabinoid system's importance as a neuromodulatory system in the brain has recently begun to surface. Neuromodulatory systems are made of several neurotransmitters which are not reabsorbed by the presynaptic neuron, and therefore spend excess time in cerebrospinal fluid modulating overall brain activity. Neuromodulators include neurotransmitters such as serotonin and dopamine, both of which play significant roles in pain perception. The brain's endocannabinoid neuromodulatory system is involved in a plethora of physiological functions related to pain, leading scientists to hypothesize that individuals with Fibromyalgia pain have dysfunctional endocannabinoid neuromodulatory systems, thus lending to their grand hypothesis that cannabinoids in cannabis bind with malfunctioning CB1 (cannabinoid receptor type 1) and CB2 (cannabinoid receptor type 2) receptors in the brain's endocannabinoid neuromodulatory system to repair malfunction and relieve pain.

After conducting a study based partly on this hypothesis, the National Pain Foundation concluded medicinal cannabis may be far more effective for treating Fibromyalgia pain than pharmaceuticals. The study compared Savella®, Lyrica®, and Cymbalta®, the top 3 FDA approved drugs currently prescribed by physicians for Fibromyalgia pain. Out of 1,300 patients only 10 percent felt Lyrica® and Savella® were "very effective," and only 8 percent reported receiving pain relief from Cymbalta®. Even more disheartening, over 60 percent of the 1,300 patients who participated in the study received no pain relief at all from the medications. However, 62 percent of patients felt cannabis was "very effective" at relieving their pain, 33 percent reported cannabis offered them mild to moderate pain relief, and only 5 percent reported cannabis offered no pain relief at all.[1]

Vaporized Cannabis for Neuropathic Pain

Problematic nerve pain from neuropathy occurs when the peripheral nerves, spinal cord, and/or brain are injured; or when the sensory system malfunctions due to the manifestation of an underlying pathological condition, such as Lyme disease, or a serious injury from a catastrophic event such as a stroke or severe spinal cord damage. Effectively managing neuropathic pain with pharmaceuticals has proven quite difficult, pushing some scientists to consider unconventional analgesics such as cannabis as possible effective alternatives for neuropathic pain relief. As it turns out, cannabis may indeed be an effective alternative for neuropathic pain relief.

According to data from a clinical trial conducted by researchers from the Davis Medical Center at the University of California, vaporized cannabis containing low amounts of THC effectively reduced neuropathic pain—even in test subjects who failed to respond to conventional methods of neuropathic pain relief. In a randomized, double-blind, placebo-controlled study, test subjects were administered cannabis with a medium dose of THC (3.53 percent), cannabis with a low dose of THC (1.29 percent), or placebo cannabis. Subjects were ordered to hold the vaporizer bag with one hand, hold the vaporizer mouthpiece in their mouth with their other hand, inhale for 5 seconds, hold the vapor in their lungs for 10 seconds, and then exhale and wait 40 seconds before inhaling again. Subjects inhaled four times over the course of 60 minutes. Out of 37 test subjects who were administered cannabis with a low dose of THC, 21 reported they received pain relief after vaporizing cannabis. Out of 36 test subjects who were administered cannabis with a medium dose of THC, 22 reported a noticeable reduction in pain levels. Based on this data, researchers concluded vaporizing cannabis with low doses of the psychoactive ingredient THC can offer pain relief from neuropathy, while minimizing the cognitive effects otherwise seen in individuals using cannabis with high doses of THC.[2]

Chapter 9

MIGRAINES

M igraines are downright excruciating and, depending on their origin, can last for months without letting up and can be a daily occurrence. Migraines in the front of your head are often associated with Candida Albicans or Bartonella, while bacteria from Lyme disease and Babesia tend to linger in the back of the head, right above the neck. Regardless, they are all equally taxing and can be nothing less than frustrating to get rid of. I remember having migraines that literally lingered for months on end before discovering cannabis could relieve the pain. I exhausted seemingly every effort to no avail—Oxycodone, Hydrocodone, Demerol, Morphine, you name it. Then, of course, I tried herbal remedies such as Feverfew and so on. However, nothing quite took the edge off the way cannabis did.

Conventional methods for migraine relief are often equipped with nasty side effects, ones which may limit your quality of life more so than the migraines themselves. The newest class of migraine drugs deemed appropriate for long term use by the FDA are the "triptans." Personally, I found while triptans did in fact relieve some of my pain, they simultaneously induced an extremely frustrating pain in my jaw and the back of my neck. Though triptans are introduced to patients as a "safe" treatment for migraines, they are often associated with undesirable side effects such as chills, sweats, weakness, or changes in mental status. These changes in mental status may be associated with "serotonin syndrome," which can prove deadly. Furthermore, changes in mentality can be dangerous for individuals who already suffer from mental conditions such as Bipolar Disorder or Schizophrenia, or who have psychiatric problems of any kind. This is concerning in regards to Lyme disease and Lyme co-infections, as Lyme disease, Bartonella, and other conditions such as Pyroluria (also commonly referred to as "HPU" or "KPU") can cause severe psychological manifestations. So, it is with great pleasure that I share the following information with you.

In 1987, an unknown mechanism was published stating that after discontinuing long-term use of cannabis, some individuals reported a spontaneous onset of severe migraines.[1] This implies cannabis was perhaps either preventing the onset of migraines for these individuals or masking their pain, explaining why they only experienced the migraines after they quit using cannabis. Further validating this theory is the well-known analgesic properties of cannabis.

The University of California in San Francisco published a study in the Journal of Neuroscience explaining how triptans work to relieve migraine pain, and how cannabis may work in a similar manner void of the negative side effects of triptans. The study showed how neurotransmitters in the body's endogenous cannabinoid system play a role in treating migraines, and explained how triptans may relieve migraines by targeting the endogenous cannabinoid system to activate the brain's endogenous canna-binoid like chemicals.[1] Therefore, it makes sense that cannabis works to relieve migraines by acting in a similar manner without causing dangerous side effects such as serotonin syndrome.

The "Ideal Drug for Migraines"

Contemplating the various pharmacological properties of an "ideal migraine drug," a medical expert, clinical and adult neu-rologist, and Assistant Professor of Medicine at a prominent university, considered all of the effects a drug would have to possess to serve as a one size fits all treatment for migraines.[2] Such effects included stimulatory activity on 5-HT1 receptors for acute pain relief, antagonistic activity on 5-HT2 receptors to relieve migraine induced nausea, ability to increase depleted endorphin levels, and inhibition of substance P (the neurotrans-mitter for sensory afferent fibers, also known as the "pain transmitter")—and all at an affordable cost. While the existence of such a medication is nothing more than a fantasy for the pharmaceutical industry, it is every bit of a reality in the world of plant medicine, as cannabis seems to meet all requirements of the "ideal migraine drug" with immaculate precision.

When using cannabis to treat your own migraines, test out dif-ferent strains and methods of use to find which works best for you. I personally reaped the most benefits from rubbing oil or salves onto my forehead or onto the back of my neck at the base of my skull, depending on which area my pain was located.

Chapter 10

MUSCLE SPASTICITY

Muscle spasticity is characterized by stiff, rigid muscles. Your muscles feel uncomfortably tight, as if you are unintentionally flexing them at all times. When I first fell ill and was still naive to the seriousness of Lyme disease and ignorant of the proper term for the symptoms of muscle spasticity, I named this symptom "Pinocchio Syndrome" because it felt as if my legs were wooden and would not bend. This term not only suited my excessively stiff legs, it also suited the sudden onset of muscle spasms and involuntary jerks of my upper and lower extremities which, to the untrained eye of an onlooker, made me appear as if I had invisible strings attached to me with a puppet master fiercely pulling them at his leisure against my will.

Rigid, sore, and cramping muscles from muscle spasticity can be unbearably painful, limit proper movement of your extremities to the point where you are hardly able to so much as make it to the restroom due to an inability to bend your legs and, worst of all, can easily steal one of the most important resources needed for a full recovery from virtually any illness: deep, restful sleep. Over the counter drugs and prescription medications often provide mild pain relief at best, and fail to adequately relieve patients of pain to a degree significant enough to make a noticeable difference in their day to day quality of life. With this in mind, it is in no way difficult to comprehend why some people who suffer from muscle spasticity are now turning to unconventional methods like cannabis to manage painful symptoms. In the book *Marijuana as Medicine: The Science Behind the Controversy*, the Institute of Medicine (IOM) claims several patients have reported noticeable improvements in sleep quality and reduced pain levels as a result of smoking cannabis.[1]

Research on cannabis use in animals with symptoms of muscle spasticity supports the idea that cannabis can act as an effective medication for managing muscle spasticity. Spasms associated with muscle spasticity are believed to stem from areas of the brain responsible for movement control, many of which are home to a wealth of cannabinoid receptor sites, leading scientists to ponder cannabis' potential for reducing uncomfortable symptoms of muscle spasticity. While it may initially seem large amounts of cannabis would prove more beneficial than small amounts at doing so, as they would provide the body with more cannabinoids and thus have a greater impact on endocannabinoid receptors located in areas of the brain where symptoms originate, results from studies on rodents showed the opposite to be true. Rodents who were administered the lowest doses of cannabis displayed a noticeably greater reduction in symptoms of muscle spasticity than those who were administered larger amounts. Humans who utilize cannabis for treatment of muscle spasticity display similar results, claiming to experience greater relief from symptoms when taking mild doses as opposed to high ones.[1]

The previous information may seem a little vague in regards to dosing, as what constitutes a "mild" or "high" dose of cannabis varies greatly depending on a wide array of factors, including tolerance, sensitivities, underlying conditions, specific strains used, methods of consumption and so on. Due to personal experience, I concur that "less is more" when using cannabis to treat muscle spasticity—at least with an active Lyme disease infection. While cannabis was effective at relieving muscle spasticity in small amounts, larger amounts often provoked a flare in symptoms of muscle spasticity.

Please note: when referring to personal use of small amounts of cannabis, I am referring to the absolute minimum amount available for consumption with the method I was using (i.e. when taking oil this meant one drop, and when vaporizing this meant one inhale), with amounts two to three times higher embodying my definition of "larger amounts" in this scenario. When using Sativa dominant strains, increasing my dosage higher than the minimum amount simultaneously increased the severity of my symptoms of muscle spasticity. Why individuals with muscle spasticity react to cannabis in this manner is unclear. However, since cannabis is a potent bactericidal and anti-microbial, a Herxheimer reaction from bacterial die-off may be part of the culprit in those with Lyme disease. Like any other herb, each individual's tolerance varies. What may be considered a small dose to one person may be considered large to another, and vice versa. Therefore, giving exact instructions as to what dosage to take would be ignorant. As always, start at the lowest dose and listen to how your body responds and adjust your dose accordingly. And also, as always, use cannabis only if it is legal in your region and only after you receive approval from your licensed physician.

Cannabis Sativa Extract in the Treatment of Spasticity

Excruciating muscle spasms ail many with illnesses such as multiple sclerosis, prompting researchers from the Neurologische Rehabilitation and MS-Abteilung of the Berner Klinik in Switzerland and the Institute for Oncological and Immunological Research in Germany to conduct a study on the efficacy of an orally administered cannabis Sativa extract in the treatment of individuals with uncontrolled spasticity linked to multiple sclerosis (MS).[2] I am referencing this study on MS induced spasticity because the symptoms of multiple sclerosis are, in many ways, strikingly similar to those of Lyme disease and Lyme disease co-infections. Conventional treatments for MS spasticity include anti-spasmodic pharmaceuticals such as baclofen, dantrolene, tizandine, and gabapentin, injections of neurotoxic agents, and surgically placed intrathecal agents. Unfortunately, these treatments are often unavailable, expensive, and cause harmful side effects. Attempting to troubleshoot these roadblocks in current treatments available for MS induced spasticity, researchers examined clinical effects of cannabis in patients with MS by comparing spasm frequency of patients with uncontrolled muscle spasticity who were administered a standardized cannabis extract to a placebo group. Gelatin capsules encasing a whole plant cannabis extract with 2.5 mg THC and 0.9 mg CBD and placebo capsules identical in appearance were used to do so. Patients took 12 capsules per day with a glass of milk—four capsules at 12 PM, four capsules in the mid-afternoon, and four capsules before bed. At the end of the study, patients who took the active cannabis containing capsules showed a decrease in the amount of muscle spasms experienced throughout the day, as well as an increase in mobility and sleep quality. It is important to note those who took a significantly higher dose of THC, as in 15 mg a day as opposed to 10 mg a day, experienced a much greater reduction in symptoms of muscle spasticity compared to other patients.

Chapter 11

MEMORY LOSS

L yme disease, Lyme co-infections, and related conditions are notorious for their tendency to induce brain inflammation, which instigates a plethora of uncomfortable symptoms. MedlinePlus, a website ran by the U.S. National Library of Medicine and National Institutes of Health, both government related organizations, claims encephalitis is rare and typically occurs only in infants and decreases with age. However, the same site also states—on the very same page—that encephalitis is caused by autoimmune diseases, Lyme disease, Syphilis, West Nile Virus, roundworms, parasites, and toxoplasmosis and other bacterial infections, as well as a lengthy list of other reasons, including iatrogenic causes such as vaccines. Even if you only consider the amount of individuals with the diseases listed above, which only account for a portion of conditions that cause encephalitis, it is difficult to fathom that "rare" is an appropriate word to use when describing encephalitis. In fact, encephalitis certainly is not rare in chronic Lyme disease—a fact that, in hindsight, makes the reason as to why encephalitis is listed as "rare" on such a site more comprehensible, considering chronic Lyme disease itself is listed as "rare" by the Centers for Disease Control. Perhaps this is done out of good intentions to prevent the public from falling into a state of panic, albeit at the risk of the dangerous consequences of acting from a source of ignorance; or perhaps there are deeper ulterior motives at play which are not in the least bit concerned with the best interest of the public.

Simply put, encephalitis is inflammation or swelling of the brain, a condition equipped with potential to display an impressively extensive laundry list of symptoms, including headaches, abnormal gait, disorientation, fatigue, sensitivity to light, stiffness throughout the body (but most commonly in the neck and/or back), rage, irritability, vomiting, muscle weakness, paralysis, loss of consciousness, seizures, short term memory loss, long term memory loss, amnesia, speech problems and more, with the worst being death. All of these symptoms may be attributed to various other conditions other than Lyme disease or Lyme induced encephalitis though.

However, if you are aware you are infected with Lyme disease or any of the above mentioned conditions which may cause encephalitis, then to say the matter should be approached seriously and with caution is to put it lightly. The grand question is, though, whether or not the symptoms listed above are from the presence of Lyme disease itself and have no association with encephalitis, or if they are manifestations of Lyme disease induced encephalitis. For me, the latter hypothesis seemed to be the case, as cannabis reduces brain inflammation and many of my symptoms matching the possible symptoms of brain inflammation either rapidly dissipated entirely or greatly lessened in severity shortly after ingesting it. Due to the acute nature of relief from almost all of the symptoms related to encephalitis, a reduction in brain inflammation from cannabis likely occurred. This makes cannabis sound like a mere band aid to mask symptoms, as opposed to a means of treatment, which may hold some validity in this case. However, also true is that it simultaneously works as an anti-fungal, anti-bacterial, and anti-microbial agent, targeting infections as well.

Interestingly, but certainly not surprisingly, research has surfaced refuting the common notion that cannabis kills brain cells and impairs memory, a notion that has been hammered in our heads for decades. To think our public education system and organizations such as D.A.R.E did not, to some degree, deceive us when teaching us about the dangers of cannabis when growing up would essentially be to not think. Thanks to brave researchers and patients who continue to come forward with evidence proving the medicinal benefits of cannabis, one is only required to possess the minutest amount of comprehensive thinking ability in order to separate fact from fiction, and reality from conditioning.

Researchers at Ohio State University found certain components of cannabis to be beneficial for the aging brain by reducing brain inflammation and regenerating dead brain cells.[1] Such information may come as an astounding fact to many, as it is the complete opposite of what we have been taught about the effects of cannabis on the brain. The common notion that cannabis use of any kind impairs memory function and kills brain cells is turning out to be quite contradictory to the truth, meaning public schools and organizations we trusted to help us were, in reality, harming us by robbing us of truths holding the potential to save our own lives and/or the lives of our loved ones. Perhaps it is most fair to say we were told "half-truths" about cannabis growing up, though, as opposed to complete lies, considering memory loss from cannabis use can occur if used excessively on a regular basis. Basically, many of you were only told one side of the story regarding the effects cannabis has on the body—until now.

This research would be an especially exciting breakthrough for those affected by Alzheimer's disease, which is thought to be the result of a chronically inflamed brain, if the government miraculously woke up and ceased to deny human beings of their right to lead healthier lives by nationally legalizing medicinal use of cannabis. Furthermore, this research offers a potentially major breakthrough for those with late stage neurological Lyme disease (neuroborreliosis) and related illnesses, as a vast majority of debilitating symptoms caused by these diseases stem from inflammation of the brain.

Due to its ability to regenerate brain cells and reduce brain inflammation, it is quite possible cannabis will be, and always has been, the perfect antidote to neurodegenerative diseases. One can only hope others will continue to bravely speak out about the benefits of cannabis in an effort to give future generations a shot at a health care system, and ultimately a quality of life, unparalleled to our own.

CB2 Receptors and Neuro-inflammatory Pathologies

As highly lipophilic molecules able to easily access the brain, cannabinoids are excellent contenders for treating pathological diseases linked to neuro-inflammation. Cannabinoids can be manipulated to target specific cannabinoid receptors in the brain, a quality extremely useful for treating brain inflammation.

Stimulation of microglial cells leads to inflammation of the brain, a process which cannabinoids may be able to halt. Activating CB2 receptors suppresses activity of microglial cells. This, along with their ability to readily penetrate the blood brain barrier, led researchers at the Virginia Commonwealth University School of Medicine to consider cannabinoids as possible contenders for abolishing neuro-inflammatory pathologies.[2] They concluded cannabinoids selectively target cells that express CB2 receptors, particularly microglial cells, enabling them to play a prominent role in neuro-inflammatory processes.

**Although you may know a habitual smoker who seems to suffer from memory loss, it is important to note that said benefits of cannabis were achieved using extremely low doses. Researchers discovered a single puff a day (research was conducted on users who smoke cannabis) is enough to provide an individual with significant, long-lasting health benefits. Still, always consult your physician before beginning this or any other new treatment.

Chapter 12

SLEEP MODULATION

*I*t does not matter what your life situation is like—whether you have Lyme disease or another illness that causes insomnia, or suffer from insomnia void of disease, of one thing I am sure: the hours you spend lying in the dark with your brain quite simply refusing to click "off" and slip into sleep, despite your every bone, every cell, every muscle, and every inch of your body desperately pleading for the replenishment only deep rest can provide, are downright excruciating. Every passing second is mentally, physically, and spiritually exhausting to the core.

Personally, I find I get little, if anything, achieved after losing a night of sleep, because there is no such thing as "not having to sleep." There is only *not* being able to sleep, and existing in that state of being diminishes every aspect of your quality of life. Add having a chronic condition to the scenario, and the consequences of failing to get adequate amounts of sleep on a regular basis are amplified tenfold. To reach remission from Lyme disease or Lyme co-infections without first overcoming insomnia is to experience a miracle, as it seems no amount of sleeping medication alleviates Lyme induced insomnia. The amount of sleeping medications I took some nights was enough to put the average individual into a medically induced coma—or at least to sleep for 24 hours. I took everything out there—Nyquil, Valerian root, Trazodone, Benadryl, Melatonin, and so on—to no avail. Nothing worked. Nothing, until I got my hands on the right strain of cannabis. While sativa dominant strains stimulated my mind and kept me awake, Indica dominant strains induced what, to me, after countless nights of staring at the wall at 3:00 A.M., was a sleep that was nothing short of heavenly.

Cannabis is a superb alternative to sleep medications for many reasons. Many medications for insomnia are unsuitable for long term use, cause undesirable side effects such as sleep walking or drowsiness the next day, are addictive in nature, and/or create a chemical dependency in users. Furthermore, they hold potential for fatal overdoses. Cannabis, on the other hand, is void of these risk factors. No fatalities from cannabis have been reported to date, and whether or not a person can become chemically addicted to it is debatable. For the sake of having an open mind, it is perhaps safer to say that cannabis use may be "habit forming," as opposed to addicting—meaning habitual use is not instigated by a chemical addiction, but by a mental one in people with addictive personalities who tend to look for any possible crutch to escape reality, whether it be cannabis or any other potentially mind altering substance readily available to them.

Improvements in sleep have been reported by at least 70 percent of people who use cannabis for medicinal purposes involving sleep disorders.[1] Cannabis helps with sleep by activating the endocannabinoid system, which can cause drowsiness when activated and is responsible for regulating the brain's sleep wake cycle. Studies show cannabis helps those who suffer from insomnia fall asleep faster and decreases sleep interruptions. Evidence from recent research supports the idea that cannabis improves sleep in those who suffer from insomnia due to pain related conditions such as fibromyalgia, multiple sclerosis, and cancer.[2] It is important to note the extent to which cannabis does or does not improve sleep quality is strongly linked to what strain of cannabis is used. Indica is ideal for sleep for the majority of people, as Sativa can be mentally stimulating. However, some people do find both Sativa and Indica beneficial for sleep.

How Cannabis Affects Sleep

As previously mentioned, cannabis interacts with the body's endocannabinoid system, which is involved in biological functions responsible for naturally regulating sleep wake cycles. Normal, healthy sleep consists of four stages grouped into two main categories, NREM sleep and REM sleep. NREM sleep is composed of stages one-three of sleep, while REM sleep is composed solely of stage four.

Stage one occurs during the initial 5-10 minutes after you fall asleep. It is characterized by a very light state of sleep, one in which you may still feel somewhat conscious. It is so light that, if woken, you will most likely believe you had never fallen asleep and were lucid the entire time. Next, the processes of stage two are set into play, as your heart rate slows and your body temperature drops. Stage two, also a relatively light state of sleep, lasts for about 20 minutes, at which point your body enters a state of deep sleep and effortlessly shifts into the third stage of sleep. Stage three is also referred to as slow-wave sleep, deep sleep, or delta sleep. During this stage, blood flow to your brain is redirected to your muscles, prompting your brain waves to slow down dramatically. Not only does redirecting blood flow in this way help you relax and enter deep sleep by relaxing your muscles and calming brain stimulation, it simultaneously restores physical energy as well, hopefully leaving you refreshed and energized upon waking. This state lasts approximately 30 minutes, at which point you enter the fourth stage of sleep, better known as REM sleep.

REM sleep is the longest stage of sleep, and is the state in which dreams occur. Rapid eye movements are a key characteristic of REM sleep, as are an increase in breathing and heart rate. Brain activity is actually increased during REM sleep, making vivid dreams possible. Although your brain activity becomes heightened, your limbs become immobilized.

Unfortunately, many who have difficulty sleeping fail to fully go through all of the sleep cycles, a process dire to healthy functioning of the body—and one of the most important factors when striving to heal. Cannabis may be the clinical pearl needed to solve this problem, as it increases the amount of time spent in stage three, or slow-wave, sleep. In doing so, it decreases the amount of time spent in REM sleep. Clearly, this fact paints cannabis' effects on sleep as negative. On the contrary, research still shows cannabis is a beneficial sleep aid because, according to sleep experts, damaging effects of sleep deprivation are primarily a result of an insufficient amount of slow-wave sleep.[3]

The Theory That Cannabis Impairs Sleep

Some researchers believe cannabis does not improve sleep, but is instead linked to sleep problems. As previously mentioned, depending on what strain is used, cannabis can either help you fall asleep or provide you with energy. So, there is some truth to this theory. The truth is never that simple, though. Abruptly quitting cannabis after steadily using it for insomnia on a long term basis may temporarily exacerbate symptoms of sleep disorders. That many people with chronic sleep problems have underlying conditions which must be addressed in order for their sleep problems to be permanently corrected should be kept in mind. If a person finds they cannot sleep after quitting cannabis, the problem could possibly be an underlying condition. After all, the sleep problems were there to begin with, which is why cannabis was implemented as a sleep aid—to reiterate: it was needed as a sleep aid. Needless to say, the jury is still out on the issue and further research needs to be conducted on it. Still, results will always vary among individuals. Like most herbs, testing the waters to see how you respond is the most foolproof method of finding whether or not cannabis helps you sleep or not. Please remember to use cannabis only if it is legal in your area, and only under the supervision of a healthcare professional.

The Effects of THC in Patients with Sleep Apnea

Sleep apnea is a common sleep disorder among patients with Lyme disease. Of the three types of sleep apnea—central sleep apnea (CSA), obstructive sleep apnea (OSA), and mixed sleep apnea (a combination of both central and obstructive sleep apnea)—obstructive sleep apnea is the most common type seen in patients with chronic, late stage Lyme disease. Obstructive sleep apnea occurs during the fourth stage of sleep, or deep sleep, prompting airways to close and resulting in an inability to exhale for, on average, approximately 20-40 seconds. Decrease in respiration (hypopnea) or a temporary complete suspension of breathing (complete apnea) may occur as a result of these involuntary pauses in breath. Low blood oxygen levels, as well as complications as serious as hypertension or even heart failure, may result due to the overwhelming amount of stress placed on the heart. Plausible explanations as to why sleep apnea is a common occurrence in individuals with Lyme disease include neurological abnormalities and dysfunction of the uvula, the small soft piece of flesh dangling downward from the middle of the soft palate in the back of the mouth. Other conditions related to Lyme disease that may cause sleep apnea include, but are not limited to, Parvovirus B19, Epstein-Barr virus, and Bartonella.

Three researchers from the department of Medicine, the department of Pharmacology, and the department of Biobehavioral Health Science at the University of Illinois executed a study on the efficacy and safety of dronabinol, a capsule containing synthesized delta-9-tetrahydrocannabinol (THC), in patients with Obstructive Sleep Apnea.[4] Their study was prompted by data from other studies on sleep apnea and THC conducted on animals suggesting that THC stabilizes autonomic output during sleep, blocks serotonin-induced exacerbation of sleep apnea, and reduces spontaneous disruptions in breathing during sleep. Rather than execute another study on THC and sleep apnea in animals, researchers used actual patients with obstructive sleep apnea. Seventeen adults with an approximate baseline Apnea Hypopnea Index (AHI), an index measuring the hourly number of pauses in breathing lasting for at least 10 seconds, of at least 15 were administered 2.5-10 mg of dronabinol daily. Results showed dronabinol, or synthetic THC, significantly reduces Apnea Hypopnea Index and is safe and well tolerated in patients with Obstructive Sleep Apnea.

As you can see, cannabis has the potential to be very helpful for treating sleep-related conditions. Many pharmaceuticals prescribed for sleep-related conditions cause unwanted side effects, such as grogginess the next day. Natural sleep-aids like cannabis that are void of the negative side effects caused by pharmaceuticals are greatly needed.

Chapter 13

PTSD AND MENTAL TRAUMA

When people think of Post-Traumatic Stress Disorder, or PTSD, they primarily associate it with individuals who have experienced extreme acute emotional trauma, such as someone in the military who experienced a bombing in war or someone who was brutally assaulted. However, a person can also develop symptoms of PTSD from trauma of mild to moderate stress that is chronic or common in occurrence, not unlike the stress experienced by those with chronic Lyme disease and other chronic and debilitating illnesses. PTSD occurs in people who go through extreme emotional trauma involving a perceived threat of death or severe injury. For people with Lyme disease and related conditions, this can happen on a daily basis, and living with a perceived threat of death or injury often becomes a way of life.

An article in the Lyme Alliance Newsletter, titled "Posttraumatic Stress Disorder and Infectious Encephalopathies," explored the association between PTSD and chronic tick-borne infections, and what effect their connection has on the human brain.[1] Two cases were presented for observation, showing PTSD is linked to an increase in the severity of symptoms experienced by individuals with chronic tick-borne infections, as well as a greater difficulty in recovering to optimal health. It was also found that emotional trauma contributes to relapses in those with infectious tick-borne illnesses. Just the same, chronic infectious tick-borne illnesses such as Lyme disease can contribute to the onset of PTSD.

The Connection between the Endocannabinoid System and PTSD

The endocannabinoid system is inextricably connected to memory functions in the brain, specifically "memory extinction." Memory extinction is the normal process of removing associations between past events and stimuli in healthy, properly functioning brains. However, this function is not properly carried out in those with PTSD, which is why they continue to respond to stimuli reminding them of the initial trauma even when such a response is no longer appropriate, or a direct threat is no longer present. In regards to Lyme disease, this can be seen in a scenario as simple as being in the same environment you were in when you first fell severely ill. For example, if you are in the same bedroom you were in when you became debilitated and have spent years of excruciating pain in that room, you are likely to associate your room with pain and perceive it as a traumatic place as opposed to one of healing. This can create negative blocks in your mind, essentially blocking you from healing entirely, or at least rendering healing a far more challenging feat than if you were in an environment that your subconscious associated with positive and healing thoughts, as you are unable to achieve the appropriate mindset needed to fully heal.

According to an Israeli scientist, cannabis might be the missing link needed for those with PTSD to recover because of its ability to aid in the process of memory extinction and ultimately diminish the brain's association between past trauma and stimuli such as certain noises, stressors, or aesthetics of the external environment.[2] An experiment conducted on mice demonstrated how cannabis does so by activating the endocannabinoid system. According to the study, animals who are electrically shocked after hearing a particular noise will forget about the shock and the trauma surrounding the noise within a few days of repeatedly hearing the noise without the initial simultaneous administration of an electrical shock. However, mice without active, properly functioning endocannabinoid systems never forget the association between the noise and the electrical shock, even when it ceases to occur with the noise. A negative block linking the noise to the trauma of the electrical shock exists indefinitely, similar to how those with PTSD continue to link stimuli to a trauma they lived through despite the passing of time.

Specifics on what strains of cannabis are best for treating PTSD have yet to be properly identified in studies. This could be because all strains are beneficial to some degree, but is most likely because studies on using cannabis to treat symptoms of PTSD were relatively nonexistent until recently. Other studies on cannabis and PTSD are still being conducted, and strain specifics will likely emerge as the results of more studies do.

In the meantime, using cannabinoids to activate the endocannabinoid system may be the key to combatting symptoms of PTSD. Since cannabinoids in general are beneficial, most if not all strains may prove useful to some extent. I suppose one would have to personally experiment with different strains of cannabis in order to find which best alleviates symptoms of PTSD.

Chapter 14

DEPRESSION

If you have Lyme disease or an associated illness, you are bound to meet, or unfortunately become, a person who wants to give up on life at some point. Unfortunately, conventional treatments for depression are often ineffective, and suicides due to Lyme disease are anything but unheard of. When someone with the same illness as you commits suicide, you empathize with their pain at the very core of your being regardless of whether you knew them personally or not; because the sting of a darkness so deep you yearn for death has most likely brushed you at least once during your own journey to reclaiming your health. You may feel hopeless and want to give up on life altogether at times—perhaps on rare occasions, perhaps more often than not, or perhaps with every breath you take. To what degree a person with Lyme disease experiences depression varies greatly, as it seems no two cases of Lyme disease and Lyme co-infections are entirely identical in nature.

However, there is one detail present among almost all cases of chronic and debilitating illnesses—eventually, the depression inflicted by these diseases exhales its darkness upon its hosts, and its breath settles in as toxic thick smog covering all that surrounds them. The toxicity of this darkness alone can seem deadly, as it can paint the illusion that you are living a waking death from which you will never return. This depression does not have to be permanent, though. Despite any failed efforts to alleviate your depression using conventional medicine, there is hope. For me, and many others, such hope resides within the healing realms of cannabis. Note to the reader: Depression is a serious and dangerous medical condition; if you suffer from depression, please seek professional medical care. This chapter is intended to share the author's experiences and opinions only.

Safety and Effectiveness of Conventional Antidepressant Medications

In the conventional medical world, telling a doctor you are suffering from depression typically results in you walking out of their office with a script for a pharmaceutical, namely a synthetic antidepressant. The most popular types of antidepressants are tricyclic antidepressants, MAOIs (monoamine oxidase inhibitors), SSRIs (selective serotonin reuptake inhibitors), and SNRIs (serotonin norepinephrine reuptake inhibitors).

Patient reports of significant relief from symptoms of depression due to antidepressant pharmaceuticals are scarce, while reports of significant increases of new symptoms from the side effects of these medications are abundant. Common side effects of tricyclics include blurred vision, constipation, brain fog, fatigue, difficulty urinating, and high blood pressure. Common side effects of MAO inhibitors include dizziness, weakness, migraines, tremors, and, if mixed with certain other drugs, fatality. SSRIs are known for causing insomnia, appetite loss, weight loss, nausea, nervousness, headaches, and sexual dysfunction. SNRIs can cause weight loss, appetite loss, fatigue, insomnia, headaches, sexual dysfunction, liver failure, and high blood pressure.

Equally alarming is the increase in suicidal thoughts and behaviors among those who take antidepressants—the very thing that was supposed to subdue suicidal tendencies may instead amplify them, a side effect seen mostly in adolescents under the age of 18. There has been debate over whether this is true or not. However, that the issue was of enough concern for Great Britain to altogether ban the use of antidepressants on patients under the age of 18, and that the FDA now requires dire warnings of this side effect on all antidepressant bottles, speaks volumes about their safety—or lack thereof. Needless to say, it is not uncommon for people to find the side effects of pharmaceutical antidepressants to be worse than the initial symptoms of depression itself. As if the side effects were not bad enough, a person must first suffer through an increase in symptoms due to withdrawals before they can rid themselves of the undesirable effects of these medications. Furthermore, residues from synthetic antidepressants bind to receptors in the brain, indefinitely—unless a person undergoes rigorous detoxification to expel the chemical residues from their body. Due to this, people who have taken these medications are typically less responsive to treatments for Lyme disease and Lyme disease co-infections; as their nutrients are unable to properly bind to their receptors, a process crucial for combating malnutrition conditions, which many infectious illnesses essentially are, especially Mycoplasma.

The Relationship between Cannabis and Depression

There is great debate over whether or not cannabis relieves depression or actually sparks onset of, or worsens severity of preexisting, symptoms of depression. Like most debates, there may be truth to both sides of this one. It is true cannabis effectively treats depression. It is also true cannabis may induce, or increase the severity of, depression. Solving this debate lies in the simple understanding that cannabis, like all other medications, manifests impressive results when used correctly, and damaging ones when used incorrectly. At low doses, cannabis can be an effective antidepressant; at higher doses, cannabis may actually increase or initiate symptoms of depression.

A neurobiological study conducted on rats by Dr. Gabriella Gobbi of McGill University showed cannabis works as a potent antidepressant when administered in relatively low amounts, but may worsen depression when administered in higher amounts.[1] To test the effects of cannabis on depression, researchers injected rats with the synthetic cannabinoid WIN55, 212-2. Next, they tested the rats for depression using the Forced Swim test—a standardized test used to measure depression in animals. Results showed cannabis to be sufficiently equipped with all necessary properties embodying the ideal mechanisms of an effectual antidepressant, as it successfully lessened symptoms of depression by increasing activity in neurons responsible for serotonin production.

According to Dr. Gobbi, the antidepressant qualities of cannabis stem from its relationship with the endocannabinoid system in the brain. By interacting with CB1 receptors, which directly impact cells that produce serotonin, cannabinoids essentially function as mood stabilizers. Dr. Gobbi's study eloquently displayed how low doses of cannabis increase levels of serotonin, the neurotransmitter in the brain that, when depleted, leads to depression. Since depression sufferers tend to have low levels of serotonin, SSRIs such as Prozac and Celexa were designed with the intention of increasing readily available levels of serotonin in the brain. Unfortunately, as peviously discussed, increasing serotonin levels via pharmacological intervention oftentimes comes at a substantial cost—further diminishment in one's quality of life, on account of the lengthy list of possible side effects of conventional antidepressants.

In conclusion, Dr. Gobbi made the following comment regarding the results of her study on cannabis and depression:

> *"Low doses had a potent antidepressant effect, but when we increased the dose, the serotonin in the rats' brain actually dropped below the level of those in the control group. So we actually demonstrated a double effect: At low doses it increases serotonin, but at higher doses the effect is devastating, completely reversed."* [1]

Chapter 15

ANXIETY

*B*efore I had firsthand experience with the healing qualities of cannabis, I clung to the belief I was conditioned to
believe since elementary school—that cannabis was a harmful
plant. I experimented with it various times, and each time I got
massive anxiety, paranoia, and my legs involuntarily twitched. Of
course, my paranoia only amplified the twitching and thus the
anxiety, because I would dwell on whether or not those around
me noticed my spasms. As it turns out, many others experience
anxiety from certain strains of cannabis. However, it is mild to
moderate and relatively short lived, compared to my severe
anxiety attacks that sometimes lasted several hours. For the
average (healthy) individual, cannabis induced anxiety typically
subsides within 30 minutes, allocating them an experience that
truly is enjoyable, or at least not incredibly terrible like mine.

Perhaps my experience with cannabis was so different than the
average individual's because, unbeknownst to me, I already had

Lyme disease by the time I tried it; and therefore had no reason to be anything but entirely oblivious to the relationship between cannabis and Lyme disease. In fact, at 16, the very idea that cannabis could be used as a medicine was foreign to me, a thought from a distant land whose winds had yet to blow my way—but most certainly would in the future. So, at the time, I simply believed I reacted differently to cannabis than others, and decided that since my reaction was so unenjoyable, I would merely ban it from my life indefinitely.

Fast forward six years, and I suddenly found myself offering prayers of extreme gratitude to the universe for providing me—for providing *us*—with cannabis. Suddenly, to me, it had become one of the most incredible, life changing medications—so much so that, within a matter of months, it did what none of the plethora of other medications I had tried during the previous two years were able to do. It gave me my life back. I quickly learned the reason my negative side effects were amplified to such a significant degree in the past was because I was already sharing my body with spirochetes; and cannabis has strong bactericidal properties, enabling it to potentially instigate an increase in symptoms due to bacterial die-off, also known as a Herxheimer Reaction. In retrospect, perhaps my horrible reactions to cannabis in the past were due to bacterial die-off and were, in reality, a good thing.

When I dove into unknown waters and began treating myself with cannabis, I honestly did not care if it caused unbearable anxiety like it had in the past. Knowledge truly is power and, for me, becoming aware of the scientific reasons for the uncomfortable or painful symptoms that presented themselves while under the influence of cannabis enabled me to snap myself out of the "I'm going to die" anxiety attacks when they did occur. Understanding the scientific explanation of things makes otherwise alarming situations endurable, as it reminds me what I am going through is a natural reaction. So, in the event that you feel the same way, I am going to attempt to briefly explain the link between cannabis and anxiety to you.

How Cannabinoids Interact with the Amygdala's Natural Endocannabinoid System to Reduce Anxiety

Cannabis has been used as an antidote to anxiety for centuries, with the first recorded account occurring in 1563, when naturalist Garcia da Orta referred to cannabis as an herb that aided anxiety laden individuals by helping them to be "delivered from all worries and care," in his publication *Colloquies on the simples and drugs of India*.[1] Of course, the validity of this statement has since been exhaustingly questioned, torn apart by conflicting reports claiming cannabis use actually causes or intensifies anxiety, resulting in extreme panic attacks, which clearly manifest anything but delivery from all of one's "worries and cares." It suffices to say the relationship between cannabis and anxiety is a great deal more intricate than Orta's description. Orta's statement regarding the ability of cannabis to reduce anxiety is true—but only part of the time. Sometimes, the exact opposite happens. Apprehension ensues and anxiety levels steadily surge, brewing a volcano whose inevitable eruption gives birth to a full blown panic attack, causing a person to wholeheartedly believe in his or her imminent death for no apparent or logical reason. I suppose a more accurate way of describing the relationship between cannabis and anxiety, if wishing to appeal to all circumstances, would be to say that cannabis can deliver a person from all worries and care depending on various factors, such as the strain and amount of cannabis used.

Despite past research linking cannabis to the onset of anxiety, depression, schizophrenia, bipolar disorder, and other mental illnesses, a study on mice conducted at Vanderbilt University in Tennessee showed cannabis reduces anxiety levels and calms the body's fight-or-flight response when taken in small doses.[2] The study was the first to ever demonstrate how nerve cells in the amygdala—the part of the brain responsible for regulating anxiety levels and the fight-or-flight-response—produce and release their own natural endocannabinoids. As a system, these natural endocannabinoids regulate fight-or-flight response, thus preventing spikes in anxiety levels by subduing the amount to which receptors in the amygdala react to overstimulation.

Numbers of natural endocannabinoids produced in the amygdala are reduced when an individual experiences chronic stress or severe psychological trauma, resulting in heightened anxiety levels. By interacting with cannabinoid receptors, cannabinoids make up for the deficiency of naturally occurring endocannabinoids in the amygdala, thereby eliminating anxiety by addressing it at the root of its manifestation. However, this is not a long term fix. Over time, cannabis can reduce the efficiency of cannabinoid receptors in the brain and paradoxically instigate anxiety instead. All in all, it seems safe to say less is always more when using cannabis to treat anxiety, regarding both references concerning "amounts" of use—the amount of cannabis consumed, and the amount of time it is consumed for.

The Relationship Between THC, CBD, and Anxiety

THC, which interacts with CB1 receptors, has paradoxical effects on anxiety, producing polar opposite results depending on the quantity administered. Low doses of THC help alleviate symptoms of anxiety, while high doses of THC amplify them. Unlike THC, CBD exhibits little to no activity with CB1 receptors. Nonetheless, CBD has proven itself as a cannabinoid fully equipped with potential to treat anxiety. One of CBD's most notable effects on anxiety is its synergistic effect with THC. In a study published in 1982, CBD displayed the ability to block anxiety instigated by THC,[3] depending on the CBD to THC ratio of the strain being used—which is to say, strains higher in CBD, such as Indica or Indica dominant strains, are more beneficial for treating anxiety than strains high in THC and low in CBD, like Sativa and Sativa dominant strains. Without enough CBD to block THC induced anxiety, Sativa and Sativa dominant strains are capable of producing anxiety ranging from merely uncomfortable to absolutely unbearable.

The Effects of CBD on Social Anxiety

Oddly, one of the hardest obstacles I faced as I began regaining my health was the process of reintegrating myself back into society, the very thing I had so desperately yearned to do in the dark of the night for well over 600 nights in a row. I never considered how spending so much time in isolation would influence my doing so. I naively assumed I would slip right back into the world as swiftly as I had slipped out of it. Unfortunately, instead of meeting new people and forming new relationships, I was met with the stark reality of what it means to have social anxiety, and the only relationship that blossomed was the one I had with it. Each time I tried to hang out with old friends, or do something work related, it seemed the only part of me that showed up was anxiety. Then again, that isn't really "me." So, I suppose it is more accurate to say anxiety possessed me, controlling my thoughts and behavior, its poison radiating to the brims of my fingertips, until all traces of my true self were hidden. When in a crowd of people, especially when I was the one speaking, the thoughts swirling about my mind were polluted with fear and anxiety. *Was I speaking correctly? Was I standing correctly? Was I using the right words? Was everyone thinking about how foolish I sounded? Surely, they were. Had anyone noticed the slight quiver to my voice? And for god's sake, was I holding my shoulders up correctly or any other body part for that matter?* Clearly, I was drowning in a pool of social anxiety.

By no means was breaking ties with social anxiety easy. Sometimes, I still struggle with it, but research and personal experience have proven CBD takes the edge off social anxiety. Of course, you could throw yourself in the opposite direction and heighten symptoms of social anxiety if a strain of cannabis with a high THC content is used. CBD oil is a great alternative to actual cannabis, as it is an isolated extract of cannabidiol, the actual cannabinoid proven to treat social anxiety; and is void of THC, the cannabinoid typically responsible for increasing anxiety. Furthermore, it is legal to purchase and use CBD oil products in most places, but always double check the legalities where you live before purchasing any product.

In a study testing the effects of CBD on social anxiety, researchers administered a simulation public speaking test (SPST) to test subjects before and after taking CBD and compared the results.[4] A SPST is basically a test designed to provoke a response in an individual with social anxiety similar to the one they would experience if they were actually speaking in public. Test results showed a decrease in anxiety among individuals treated with CBD, with the placebo group presenting much higher levels of anxiety, cognitive impairment, discomfort, and alertness in comparison. Preliminary findings of the study, published in the *Neuropsychopharmacology journal* under the title "Cannabidiol Reduces the Anxiety Induced by Simulated Public Speaking in Treatment-Naive Social Phobia Patients," indicate that as little as a single dose of CBD can drastically reduce social anxiety and related symptoms, such as cognitive impairment, difficulties in speech delivery, and frantic, anticipatory speech. Not only did CBD ease the process of speaking for test subjects, but, due to improved speaker performance, it enhanced the audience's attention as well—rendering speeches delivered by those who were administered CBD before speaking as all around more productive than those delivered by speakers who were not administered CBD. Simply put, the simulation public speaking test revealed that CBD inhibits one of the most prominent symptoms of social anxiety, fear of public speaking.

Other interesting details surfaced as an outcome of the study, though. After administration of CBD, MRI scans of those with social anxiety revealed CBD provokes action in the limbic and paralimbic brain areas, which are both linked to anxiety. Another notable effect of CBD on social anxiety seen in the study was its ability to almost entirely eliminate thoughts of negative self-evaluation while speaking in individuals whose minds would have usually ripped everything they said to shreds as they spoke, convincing them they were doing a horrible job, due to limiting thoughts and beliefs typically inflicted upon them by intense social anxiety.

Why Anxiety from Cannabis Use May Be More Severe in those with Lyme Disease

Many who use cannabis admit to having at least one bad experience with the herb in the past, in which they succumbed to extreme anxiety and/or paranoia. However, it is important to understand the cannabis induced episodes of anxiety that many of these people are referring to are quite subtle compared to those experienced by individuals with Lyme disease. Why is this so? Many with chronic Lyme disease live in a constant state of "fight or flight," the body's defense mechanism to a perceived threat. For this to occur, the amygdala is activated and there is an increase in the amount of the adrenaline, norepinephrine, and cortisol released in the body—all of which generate anxiety. So, for a person with Lyme disease who already has an overactive amygdala, anxiety from the increased release of these adrenal hormones is amplified, as they already have an excessive amount of these hormones soaring throughout their bodies.

So, What Can You Do?

There are a few options. First, you can realize the reason for the intense anxiety you feel after using cannabis is from an increase in adrenaline and cortisol levels due to THC's relationship with the amygdala, meaning the feelings of panic and paranoia you are experiencing will fade. In other words, that you are dying is a false illusion created by your mind that will dissipate with time, along with any other anxiety induced thoughts or symptoms. Another option, of course, is to utilize pure CBD oil which is void of the psychoactive agent THC, the primary component in cannabis responsible for causing anxiety. However, I find it important to note that it may be significantly less beneficial to attempt to utilize cannabis as a bactericide without THC or other cannabinoids. **Here's why:** Pure cannabis, as opposed to CBD oil, is far more effective as an antibacterial. CBD oil consists of cannabidiol, only one of five major cannabinoids in cannabis that displays potent activity in treating drug resistant strains of bacteria. Research has proven four other cannabinoids in cannabis—cannabichromene, cannabigerol, tetrahydrocannabinol, and cannabinol—exhibit significant antibacterial properties as well. It is true CBD oil extracted from cannabis is beneficial for treating many infections, but it is also true that using actual cannabis is potentially four times as powerful at doing so.

A quick reminder on cannabis strains and chemical makeup: As you are most likely aware, there are many, many hybrid strains of cannabis, composed of a combination of the two main species of cannabis—Indica and Sativa (there is a third species, C.Ruderalis, but its use is far more rare). Indica has a chemical makeup containing moderate amounts of both THC and CBD (one of the most commonly known cannabinoids, Cannabidiol). Sativa, on the other hand, has a chemical makeup composed of high levels of THC and low levels of CBD. For anxiety's sake, avoiding Sativa or Sativa dominant strains is preferable because THC, the psychoactive ingredient in cannabis consisting in high amounts in Sativa and Sativa dominant strains, is strongly associated with feelings of paranoia and anxiousness because it activates the fear control center of the brain, the amygdala.

Remember that anxiety can be a serious condition; please consult a licensed physician before using cannabis.

Chapter 16

SEIZURES AND CONVULSIONS

"Get it out of me, get it out of me. It is shooting sharp pains up my arm to my heart, and my entire arm is starting to go numb. Take it out, please," I pathetically begged, as a nurse looked at me both dumbfounded and ignorantly amused (the two really are not much different I suppose). This was one of my first trips to the Emergency Room post Lyme disease infection, and it proved eventful to say the least.

"It's a saline I.V. You cannot have a bad reaction to it. It can't hurt you," she said, smirking at me.

"Perhaps she genuinely thinks I am being a hypochondriac and is trying to help me lighten up, I doubt she is so incredibly bored she wants to antagonize me over, what was most likely to her, an outlandish claim—that the saline I.V. was making half my body go numb, and sending unbearable

sharp, stinging pains shooting up my left arm into my heart,"
I thought, "or perhaps, I really am being over dramati..."

She cut me off before I finished that last thought, saving me the trouble of spinning lies to myself. Squeezing the still almost full saline bag into my IV with all her might, she glared down at me, as if she was proud to be making a point of some sort—most likely the one confirming I was a hypochondriac, due to her previous condescending riddled statement on how saline could in no way hurt me. Before she could make her point, and before I could so much as care whether or not she understood mine, the numbness—perhaps more accurately described as a sort of temporary paralysis of motor neurons but not sensory neurons, as I could not move but I could feel the sensation of a thousand needles under my skin—in my arm spread throughout every limb, every muscle, every vessel, every vein in my body, from the ends of my toes to the crown of my head. The stinging pain I felt minutes prior was minute compared to the one beginning to radiate up my arm, straight into my heart. Screaming was out of the question, not only because a scream could never do the nails on a chalkboard type of disgust provoked by such a sensation justice, but because I could not speak. Even my face was numb, its muscles paralyzed, leaving me trapped in silence inside a body screaming with pain. Soon, I was no longer trapped, as I faded out of consciousness, into the dark depths of peaceful rest. When my consciousness snapped back into my body, it was ripped from the depths of peaceful rest just as rapidly as it was first ripped from the prison of my body. All I could do was laugh, but not literally, not out loud, only to myself. The joke was on me, or should I say in me? I opened my mouth to laugh, or so I thought, and nothing moved. I lifted my left arm to get my partner's attention, but only in my imagination. My mind and body, although reunited, remained simultaneously unattached.

Little by little, I came to. I slowly regained control of my body, with the left side taking significantly longer to recover. Apparently, after I went unconscious, I had a massive seizure. The nurses still did not seem to care much, though. I was sent home with a diagnosis of hypothyroidism (wait, what?), which did not so much as begin to address the symptoms that brought me to the Emergency Room, not to mention the ones that manifested while there, namely a seizure. Once home, I studied the prescription given to me by a doctor who, after visiting my bedside for well under 5 minutes, somehow felt he had gathered enough knowledge of my medical history and current state to instruct me to take a pharmaceutical thyroid medication—indefinitely. That night, returning home from the hospital, a dense fog of emotionally anesthetizing acceptance permeated within. It was a type of internal numbness, a deep feeling of desensitization, that would not leave me and would become a part of me for years to follow, and that would become, for the most part, the only consistent company I had throughout those years, welcome or not. For better or worse, that numbness, the one in which I accepted my situation without attaching emotion to it, is what enabled me to overcome so many difficult times. I was not defeated from the experience of my first seizure. Rather, I clicked into survival mode. Although seemingly slightly twisted, adopting a sense of apathy, of not feeling, allowed me to endure what was to come. What came was a tsunami of the mind, body, and soul. Included in the makings of the storm were daily seizures, sometimes up to ten an hour. **Note: This only worked for so long. I do not condone the act of not feeling in the least bit, because in retrospect, I realize the decision to not feel the bad also deprived me of the experience of feeling fully alive.

Before 400 B.C., when Hippocrates deemed epilepsy a disorder of the brain, people believed demons or gods inhabited the bodies of those with epilepsy. Fortunately, we are no longer persecuted for having seizures, at least not to the same degree as those before 400 B.C. were. Some still unfortunately endure persecution for seizures to a minor degree, though. Those of which I speak are primarily those with seizures not considered epileptic from illnesses not widely recognized by mainstream medicine, such as Lyme disease, Bartonella, Babesia, Toxoplasmosis, and Mycoplasma, just to name a few. Since seizures induced by these illnesses often display different characteristics than typical epileptic seizures, those who experience them are frequently told their seizures are not real, they are faking it, and ultimately, they are "crazy" and need to see a psychiatrist. For years, I was one of those people, with seizures so violent even 10 mg of Lorazepam (Ativan) could not control them.

After years of enduring multiple seizures a day, I finally underwent a three day EEG study which determined I did in fact have epilepsy, left temporal lobe epilepsy to be specific. However, these tests also concluded that not all of my seizures were epileptic. According to the self-proclaimed Lyme literate neurologist overseeing my studies, some of my seizures were "fake," and could only be treated by a psychiatrist. She held zero interest in discussing their possible relationship to Lyme disease or other associated conditions, perhaps because she also held zero deep-rooted knowledge on the subject. Unfortunately, ignorance is always only bliss on one side of an issue. The other side, the one that has stepped out of ignorance's dingy umbrella, the one that was me in this case, is dealt a heavy blow at the expense of the other party's delusional perceived "bliss." The notion that I was faking my seizures infuriated me, as I knew it to be, with every ounce of my being, both ridiculous and exempt of the slightest trace of validity. The seizures which they referred to as fake were ones that occurred when a strobe light was placed directly in front of my face and turned on in a dark room, in an attempt to induce a seizure and capture my brain waves during it on the

EEG machine. While I did react to the strobe lights, apparently convulsing and making odd noises, my brain waves showed no significant activity. This resulted in the doctor immediately concluding the convulsions were within my control, and that the reason I reacted physically to the strobe light was because I subconsciously knew people with epilepsy are sensitive to overstimulation, such as that of flashing lights. So, I left the hospital with two diagnoses: real seizures, and fake seizures. Later, I found out my "fake" seizures were actually possible reactions to over stimulation, and very real ones at that, due to conditions I was previously unaware I had such as HPU/KPU, or Pyroluria.

Over the years, I have been placed on alarmingly high doses of seizure medications, including outrageous, tranquilizing amounts of Lamictal and Ativan (i.e. 10+ mg a day). Regardless of the dose, no medications were able to completely control or prevent the seizures I had on a daily, oftentimes hourly, basis. Going more than two days without a seizure always felt like a miracle worthy of explosive celebration. Once I started smoking cannabis, I went ten days without a seizure, then twenty, then months, and so on. Somewhere along the way, I switched from smoking cannabis to healthier methods of intake, such as oil and edibles. If I had an aura and felt a seizure coming on, I found I could place a few drops of cannabis infused coconut or olive oil under my tongue and the aura would typically subside relatively quick, with no presence of a seizure or seizure like activity ever manifesting afterwards, minus the initial aura.

Before I started controlling my seizures with cannabis, I could not drive, go out in public for long, walk much because I had too many concussions from falling and hitting my head due to seizures, and I definitely could not go anywhere where there were loud sounds or bright lights, meaning I could not participate in outings as seemingly small as going to see a movie at the theater or out to dinner at a restaurant. By controlling my seizures, cannabis opened long shut doors allowing me to once again live the type of richly inhabited and ensouled life I forgot existed. It allowed me to drive again, to go to movies again, to enjoy concerts again, and so much more. Essentially, it returned parts of my life to me that had sailed out to sea and sunk to the bottom years ago, ones I was unsure I would ever enjoy again, so much so I had forgotten what they even felt like. In many ways, I had forgotten what it meant to feel alive. When you forget how something feels, it is impossible to miss it, making it easy to forget what you are fighting for. By controlling my seizures, cannabis blessed me with the chance to do things, to feel things, which I had not done or felt in years.

Anticonvulsant properties of cannabis are among the most ancient of its known medicinal benefits. Ancient societies of China, Africa, India, Greece, and Rome utilized cannabis as an antiepileptic and anticonvulsant. Written testimonies of the effectiveness of cannabis as an antiepileptic and anticonvulsant were recorded in western scientific journals as early as the 19th century, including the infamous one by Dr. William Brooke O'Shaughnessy on the uses of cannabis in India, published in 1860 by the Ohio Medical Society.[1] O'Shaughnessy's popularity in the field of medicinal cannabis began decades prior, though. In 1839 he did more than enter the scene of medicinal cannabis—he created it, by introducing information on the medical applications of cannabis to [then] modern Western medicine.

Little was understood about the medical properties of cannabis throughout England and Europe prior to 1839, when O'Shaughnessy lectured to a group of scholars and students at the Medical and Physical Society of Calcutta on the history of medicinal cannabis use in India and the Middle East. Although an avid advocate for the herb's use as a medicine, especially as an anticonvulsant, O'Shaughnessy did not fail to caution against taking or administering doses high enough to induce inebriation. He advised doctors to proceed with caution in treating patients with cannabis, starting with the lowest possible dose of the herb to avoid adverse reactions, and then adjusting the dose to fit each individual case. In his own words: Clinical studies [have] "led me to the belief that in hemp [cannabis] the profession has gained an anticonvulsive remedy of the greatest value."[1]

In present day society, use of cannabis as an anticonvulsant remains a subject of great debate among scientists. There is far more clarity among individual reports of its effectiveness in treating seizures and convulsions than there is in scientific literature. Many individuals with grand mal seizures claim smoking cannabis is more effective than pharmaceuticals at treating epileptic episodes and convulsions, entirely preventing the onset of any seizures in some cases. Others report cannabis reduces symptoms of seizures and convulsions, most notably by preventing a loss in consciousness when episodes occur. Some feel cannabis works best at preventing seizures and convulsions when used in conjunction with other anticonvulsants. Such individuals claim using either cannabis or their medications alone does not control their seizures at all, or at least not as effectively as taking them together does.

Anticonvulsant Effects of Cannabidivarin-Rich Cannabis Extracts

In a 2013 study published in the *British Journal of Pharmacology*, titled "Cannabidivarin-rich cannabis extracts are anticonvulsant in mouse and rat via a CB1 receptor-independent mechanism," researchers observed anticonvulsant properties of cannabis-derived botanical drug substances that were rich in cannabidivarin

(CBDV) and contained cannabidiol (CBD) using mice and rats.[2] A CBDV substance containing delta-9-tetrahydrocannabinol and delta-9-tetrahydrocannabivarin was tested, alongside a purified extract of CBDV void of psychoactive ingredients.

The unpurified CBDV botanical drug substances displayed significant anticonvulsant characteristics in two seizure models, the pentylenetetrazole and audiogenic seizure models, and inhibited pilocarpine induced convulsions. However, the anticonvulsant effects of purified CBDV and CBD drug substances were not as significant. In conclusion, the delta-9-tetrahydrocannabinol and delta-9-tetrahydrocannabivarin in the unpurified CBDV substance allotted greater rapport with CB1 cannabinoid receptors than the purified version of CBDV and CBD.

As you can see, cannabis holds promise for treating seizures. Of course, there are many different types of seizures, and what works for one person may not work for another. However, in my experience, I have found pharmaceuticals to be extremely ineffective at controlling Lyme induced seizures, as have others. So, the discovery of natural treatment options for seizures, such as cannabis, offers hope for many.

Chapter 17

RAGE

"Maybe if you wouldn't have naively pushed me on the first LLMD [Lyme Literate Medical Doctor] you found and allowed him to place me on ungodly amounts of mind altering substances, I would not be half as sick as I am now. Maybe if you were intelligent enough to so much as GOOGLE the prescriptions you generously fed to me several times a day when I was barely coherent, I would have already healed," I yelled at my mother as we sat down to dinner one evening.

I did not care that we were in a restaurant where others could hear us, and I certainly had no regard for the fact that the prescriptions I was placed on when I first fell ill were not at all my mother's fault, that she had no intention of harming me. She was frightened. I, her youngest child and only daughter, had contracted a terrifying disease she knew little if anything about, and everything about the first Lyme literate doctor she took me to suggested he was the magician who could miraculously cure me of all ailments—wishful thinking, I know. My mother was desperately trying to save my life when she took me to the first LLMD I ever saw, and I did not care as I yelled at her that day. All I cared about in my moment of rage was dismantling the truth with a monument of lies.

Honestly, I do not remember what I said next, because I spit a record amount of outrageous insults out in such a short amount of time, and therefore cannot even come close to remembering all the hurtful things I said—perhaps because I subconsciously do not want to remember myself as a monster destroying one of the people I love most, or perhaps I truly cannot remember due to a lapse in memory. My rage steadily marched on, with words spewing from my lips so fluently and methodically you would believe I truly meant them. And the truth is, the "I" who was speaking truly did mean them, because it was a different "I" than the person I am now. One drilling through my brain, void of any heart. I was a parasite, intolerable beyond belief. Tears began to fill my mother's eyes. She was trying to keep them at bay, but one insult too many allotted tears with a toxic concentration of hopelessness to pour out the corners of her eyes. This did not make me stop, as one would expect. No, it only fueled my fury more. It egged me on. Eventually, I ran out of the restaurant in an uncontrollable rage, making my way through the woods behind it until my partner caught up with me and stopped me. I entirely forgot he was even there while verbally attacking my mother. I forgot anyone was there other than her. With laser focus, my sole intent was to destroy her that day. I will never know why, and with every step I took for months following that gloomy evening, until my rage finally began to diminish, shame followed me like a shadow, its presence never falling far behind.

There is anger, and then there is blood curdling madness, a force whose only objective is to obliterate everything in its path. For a while, I was that madness. I suppose the average person would find it embarrassing to tell the previous story about themselves. To me, it is not embarrassing. It was my reality, and by reality I mean I was so far from it that the parasites hijacking my thoughts were dwelling in what was once my reality, making it theirs while smothering the real me deep beneath their existence. Just as quickly as the rage came, though, it would leave. From the outside looking in, one would easily suspect my behavior was linked to a mental condition like Bipolar disorder, requiring a psychiatrist for treatment. To those I would say: Give it whatever title makes you happy. The truth is, you could diagnose my behavior as anything in the world. Regardless of its label, only one treatment possessed the ability to rise to the occasion and control my rage as I treated the underlying cause, which was that of Lyme disease and co-infections. It was not the consciousness of a psychiatrist, a doctor of any sort, or a human being at all for that matter. Rather, it was the consciousness of a plant, whose essence soothed me and grounded me when every bit of whom I knew myself to be on a mental, physical, and spiritual level was ripped to shreds.

Many claim cannabis impairs the mind. Perhaps if used irresponsibly, like all things, it does. But for those of us who use it for one of its primary intended purposes for living, to heal and give life, it brings us back to ourselves. It takes us *out* of our impaired mental states, allowing us to lead mentally healthier lives. Everyone is deserving of well-being on every level, including psychologically. Unfortunately, it is not always a substance that is responsible for impairing the mind, or for endorsing internal and external destruction. Sometimes, it is the human mind in itself, refusing to open its doors of perception and consider all aspects of an issue. In this case, all aspects of the issue at hand include both the people who are negatively impacted by cannabis as well as those who are positively impacted by it. It is unfair to cater to the negative stigma surrounding cannabis that society has conditioned us to believe, and in turn entirely disregard those whose lives may be changed or saved if allowed to use it for medicinal purposes, in a responsible manner. It is incomprehensible, a line of thought exempt from logic and reasoning, to place more attention on those who are using cannabis for what many perceive to be the wrong reasons than on those whose lives can be dramatically improved, if not saved, by it. At some point, we must stop living from a source of fear, and begin living from one of truth, logic, and above all empathy. The evolution of mankind depends on it.

The Effects of Cannabis on Limbic Rage Syndrome, or Episodic Dyscontrol Syndrome

Also sometimes referred to as Episodic Dyscontrol Syndrome, Limbic Rage Syndrome is a seizure-like disorder originating in the limbic system. Characterized by unpredictable and seemingly unprovoked episodes of rage, which appear irrational and psychological in nature to observers, Limbic Rage is substantially misunderstood, misdiagnosed, mislabeled, undertreated, and its existence is widely unaccepted by conventional medicine. Small environmental changes and unexpected external stimuli can trigger limbic rage. Similar to auras experienced by epileptics prior to a seizure, certain symptoms may present themselves upon the onset of limbic rage, immediately prior to the actual episode of rage itself, including hallucinations and other olfactory, gustatory, visual and auditory disturbances. Those who spend a significant amount of time in the presence of an individual with limbic rage note they are often able to identify the onset of a limbic rage episode when the individual begins to display the previously mentioned symptoms of a limbic rage aura, especially with the presence of intense anxiety. Episodes of rage can last anywhere from a few minutes to a few hours, during which the afflicted individual is impossible to subdue or reason with.

Although Limbic Rage Syndrome is considered a "seizure-like" disorder, I am including it in the chapter on rage as opposed to the previous chapter on seizures and convulsions because, in many cases, it may very well be the root cause of what is typically referred to as "Lyme rage" or "Bartonella Rage." It is believed that mood swings from Lyme disease and Bartonella, particularly those characterized by periods of acute fervent rage, are possibly, in reality, not mood swings at all. Rather, they may be seizures originating deep in the limbic system, or more precisely, from deep in the part of the temporal lobe located in the limbic lobe. The limbic lobe is the part of the limbic system consisting of parts of the frontal, parietal, and temporal lobes.

Bartonella and Lyme disease affect the Limbic system in various ways. Both Bartonella and Lyme disease can cause limbic encephalitis. When the limbic system becomes inflamed, irrational episodes of fiery rage may ensue. Individuals with Lyme disease, primarily those with neurological Lyme disease (neuroborreliosis), develop overactive deep limbic systems. This makes them highly sensitive and intolerant to stress, oftentimes even in infinitesimal amounts. Over activity in the limbic system deep inside the brain triggers a release of various signals throughout the brain, prompting various possible symptoms within a person, including anxiety, panic, and hallucinations, all of which, when combined with over activity in brain waves in the deep limbic center of the brain, have a very high probability of precipitating seizure-like episodes. However, they are not commonly referred to as seizures since they present themselves as intense outbursts of rage as opposed to convulsions, episodes of staring into space involuntarily, or other characteristics typically associated with seizures. While Limbic Rage Syndrome is considered a "seizure-like" disorder, receiving a proper diagnosis of such seizures is rare because, in the case of Lyme disease, as well as other cases of Limbic Rage Syndrome, activity occurs deep in the limbic system where EEGs lack the ability to detect electrical activity. In a study of repeated depth and surface EEG studies, seizures occurring in the part of the temporal lobe located deep in the limbic center of the brain remained undetected.[4] Due to this, many are sent home from the hospital with the same frustrating words they have heard from doctors a dozen times before that go something along the lines of, "your seizures aren't real. You are faking them. Your condition is purely psychological. See a psychiatrist."

During times like this, doing more than feeling the nudges of your intuition, but following them as well, is essential. Contrary to popular belief in the world of conventional western medicine, I wholeheartedly believe you alone know if what you are suffering from is psychological in nature or if it stems from a deeper problem which a psychiatrist can only, at best, ease the amount to which you suffer from, but not actually entirely rid you from on a long term basis. For me, there was always a deep knowing that I was not crazy; and that what I was experiencing was beyond my control, requiring intervention on a deeper level than a psychiatrist could offer me. In my opinion, a person does not suddenly begin to manifest severe psychological symptoms overnight—whether it be rage, hallucinations, delusions, or any other erratic and psychotic like behaviors and tendencies. Knowing I had grown up void of rage, hallucinations, and delusions, and that their onset occurred rapidly *after* contracting Lyme disease and Lyme disease co-infections told me it was highly likely I was not insane, I was not a lost cause, and I shouldn't give up. Perhaps most importantly, it reminded me when it really comes down to it, I am my own healer. I am my own physician. I always have been, and I always will be. With that in mind, I began testing different alternative treatments to subdue my episodes of rage and the bizarre symptoms occurring before them. To date, low dose cannabis oil made from an Indica dominant strain has proven to be the only foolproof method of treatment for me. Of course, everyone is different.

Cannabinoids owe their exceptional ability to treat Limbic Rage Syndrome to their effects on dopamine in the brain. The endocannabinoid system increases availability of dopamine, a neurotransmitter serving as an "off" switch for the brain. Low dopamine levels in the brain pave the way for the opening of too many neural channels, thereby exposing the midbrain and cerebral cortex to an overwhelming amount of stimuli. By releasing dopamine from dopamine transporters, cannabinoids essentially decrease sensory input stimulation to the limbic system, and prevent overstimulation of the amygdala.

Chapter 18

STRESS

S tress can make you sick or, as it did in my case, significant-ly worsen symptoms from an already existing illness—a fact that, instead of pushing me to become more disciplined in adopting stress relief tactics, only stressed me out further. Throughout my first year with Lyme disease, I frequently found myself extremely stressed over the fact that I should not be stressed. So desperate were my attempts to entirely rid my life of stress, that I stressed myself out to a grotesque degree. During my second year of battling Lyme disease, my habit of stress-ing over not being stressed began to lessen, until it eventually became non-existent. For this to happen, I only had to change one thing about my health routine, and changing that one thing ultimately changed everything. I quit antibiotic treatment and began tapering off other pharmaceuticals I had been placed on, and instead opted for medicinal herbs, eventually including cannabis. I strongly feel quitting antibiotic treatment in general and switching to an herbal protocol, with or without cannabis, lended to this change in my physiology and thus my psychology, essentially rendering the possibility of me fully healing plausible for what I believe to be the first time. However, while it is true the herbal protocol I adopted (Stephen Buhner's protocol, to be exact) provided me a greater sense of harmony in a long term sense, it was cannabis that provided me immediate stress relief, which in many ways enabled other herbs to work to the best of their abilities by calming me and preventing unnecessary symptom flares due to stress.

Studies show cannabis can sufficiently relieve both acute and long term stress. This is good news for anyone who struggles with stress, but perhaps even more so for those who have chronic illnesses such as Lyme disease and associated conditions. Lyme disease alone creates inflammation in the body, which makes you more susceptible to catching other infections. Since stress also causes inflammation, it amplifies your already increased risk of catching other illnesses. Aside from inflammation, stress exacerbates a myriad of other symptoms including depression, anxiety, fatigue, and neurological symptoms. Chronic stress impedes spatial and working memory, thus negatively affecting the prefrontal cortex and hippocampal functioning, resulting in impairment of cognitive abilities. Studies suggest chronic stress impacts endocannabinoid levels in the brain, deeming cannabinoids as potential contenders for neutralizing and/or reversing the negative effects stress places on the brain.

The Effects of Cannabis on Acute Stress

Results of a study conducted by researchers at the Department of Psychology at the University of Haifa in Israel on the effects of cannabis on acute stress showed cannabinoids prevent negative repercussions of acute stress on the brain, particularly in areas associated with learning and memory.[1] Negative effects of acute stress on emotional learning were prevented when cannabinoid receptors were activated in the basolateral amygdala using a CB1 and CB2 receptor agonist called WIN55,212-2, a synthetic cannabinoid that produces effects similar to naturally occurring cannabinoids such as THC, but is composed of an entirely different chemical structure. This specific CB1 and CB2 receptor agonist also prevented stress related increases of corticosterone levels and stress related variations in hypothalamic-pituitary-adrenal negative feedback.

The Effects of Cannabis on Chronic Stress

Researchers at the Complutense University in Spain conducted a study on lab rats to test the efficiency of cannabis as a natural medication for stress relief.[2] According to results, activation of CB2 receptors markedly decreases inflammation induced by chronic stress. Although CB2 receptors are powerful enough to meticulously modulate immune cell activity when activated and functioning properly, they do not provoke psychoactive effects in the brain as CB1 receptors do. This suggests future production of a cannabis derived stress reliever void of the mind altering "high" frequently sparked by cannabis use, or any of the other numerous physically and mentally altering side effects of currently available pharmaceutical treatments for stress, is a feasible possibility. Dr. Garcia-Bueno, who headed the study, concluded cannabis has an "anti-inflammatory profile for CB2 receptor activation," making it of potential benefit "for the treatment of stress-related pathologies with a neuroinflammatory component, such as depression." [2]

Chapter 19

ADHD

P eople everywhere were relieved when the Ritalin craze in America subsided. Of course, it was not so much the Ritalin trend that subsided. Rather, use of the name itself faded and was replaced with a new designer drug, Vyvanse.[1] All the rage over Ritalin was, at its core, directed more towards the dangerously stimulating effects of the substance, rather than the particular brand name of the drug itself. So, a new, just as intense, medication was created under a different name and pharmaceutical companies nationwide effortlessly obtained their wish—an end to the growing hysteria over Ritalin use, and a steady rise in sales of ADHD medication.

It is an absolute myth that the FDA approves amphetamine derived substances sharing a molecular structure similar to that of the street drugs cocaine and meth (amphetamines) in medications used to treat ADHD. Quite shockingly, this is unfortunate news compared to the alternative, also known as the truth, which is considerably worse: The FDA has in fact approved the use of pure methamphetamine in ADHD medications. No longer is a substance "similar" to methamphetamine the main or only threat posed by ADHD medications, but actual methamphetamine in itself. Initially, one would think this could not possibly be true, as exposure of such information would surely provoke resistance from the general public against the medical community. And that's just it, actually. One would think, including the FDA. As a result, the mechanical, and debatably deceptive, collective minds behind the FDA instead presented the medical world with Desoxyn—a mere synonym for methamphetamine. While Desoxyn is different from street meth in some ways, it is also very similar in other ways.

While studies show the brain is able to adapt to stimulant ADHD medications over time, they also show the brain grows a tolerance to such medications at a rate proportional, at the least, to the rate at which it adapts to the drugs. Once the maximum dose of the medication ruled appropriate by the FDA is reached, as it oftentimes is when the drug is used for a long period of time (i.e. typically over the course of one year, but less in some individuals), patients frequently find themselves desolate and abandoned at the crossroads of an addiction they unconsciously and naively stumbled into. In general, this crossroads has two possible paths to choose from. One leads to addiction of stronger doses of stimulant medications obtained illegally off the street, particularly illegal stimulants such as cocaine and methamphetamines in this case. The other path involves a possible intervention and rehab, with a promise of intolerably irritating withdrawal symptoms along the way. A successful journey down this path is often highly dependent on the individual's support system, or lack thereof.

If you developed an addiction to ADHD medications you were prescribed, particularly stimulants, due to the chronic fatigue often associated with Lyme disease and associated conditions, do not feel guilty, hopeless, or so much as a drop of shame. Speaking from firsthand experience, I can attest you are far from alone. Although it may currently seem unfathomable, you possess the power to break free of the prison of stimulant addiction. After all, if you are battling a chronic illness such as Lyme disease or another similar condition, look at the insurmountable amount of struggles you have overcome in the past that you never dreamed you would be strong enough to rise above. Tools are available to aid you in the process, and to the disbelief of many—although it is highly unlikely you are among that majority if you have made it this far in a book of this nature—studies show cannabis helps cure addiction to stimulants. This particular study will be included at the end of this chapter for any who may find it useful. What's more, is that cannabis can also serve as a treatment for ADHD.

The Relationship between Cannabis, ADHD, the Endocannabinoid System, and Dopamine

Despite its infamous reputation for impairing focus in recreational users, cannabis often has the opposite effect on those with ADHD. However, the extent to which it does so is highly dependent on the said individual, in conjunction with the particular strain that is used. Those with ADHD have elevated levels of anandamide, an endogenous cannabinoid neurotransmitter released in the body as a protective response to symptoms of various stress factors, including ADHD, in an attempt to prevent the harmful effects such factors can have on the body. Coincidentally, anandamide and THC share a few key characteristics. Not only do they bind to the same cannabinoid receptors in the body, but their effects on the body are markedly similar in nature as well. As a result, researchers believe targeting the endocannabinoid system with cannabis may successfully manage symptoms of ADHD.

An inadequate level of dopamine is believed to be one of the primary root causes of ADHD. Stimulants are prescribed to treat ADHD for this reason, as they increase dopamine levels. However, stimulants are loaded with negative side effects, resulting in a great demand for an effective alternative treatment for ADHD. While there are existing alternatives for ADHD treatment other than pharmaceutical stimulants, most are not nearly as effective or powerful. Cannabis may be the missing link needed to sufficiently supply such a demand, as increasing activity in the endocannabinoid system increases dopamine release. Certain strains of cannabis, with the proper chemical profiles required to adequately increase dopamine levels to an extent great enough to relieve symptoms of ADHD, can naturally treat ADHD without placing users at risk of the laundry list of negative side effects accompanying prescription ADHD medications, such as increased heart rate, heart palpitations, cardiac arrest, high blood pressure, addiction, and excess buildup of toxic chemicals in the body from repetitious substance use.

In an interview with MSNBC, Dr. Claudia Jensen used simple logic and reasoning to explain why cannabis should be seriously considered as a treatment for ADHD, based on her clinical background as a pediatrician and her experience as an instructor at the University of Southern California[2]:

> *"They don't have to get stoned—it's dose related. But they do get the benefit of being able to focus, not be impulsive, not be angry, be peaceful and relaxed and pay attention in school, which helps them get better grades."*

Cannabis May Cure Addiction to Stimulants

"A growing number of studies support a critical role of the ECBS and its modulation by synthetic or natural cannabinoids in various neurobiological and behavioral aspects of stimulant addiction. Thus, cannabinoids modulate brain reward systems closely involved in stimulant addiction, and provide further evidence that the cannabinoid system could be explored as a potential drug discovery target for treating addiction across different classes of stimulants."—U.S. Natural Library of Medicine National Institutes of Health

In a study published by the National Institute of Health, researchers discovered cannabinoids affect the brain's reward system, which includes the components of an individual's brain responsible for determining their behavior and the amount of pleasure they feel in response to a substance, in a manner similar to that of stimulants.[3] Evidence suggests the endocannabinoid system (ECBS) can produce neurological processes similar to ones present in the brains of individuals addicted to stimulants. Researchers at The Psychiatry Research Unit at Centre Hospitalier de Montreal in Canada claim this discovery opens the door for further exploration regarding the possibility of the endocannabinoid system as a "potential drug discovery target for treating addiction across different classes of stimulants."

It is no secret that amphetamine addiction only continues to steadily and dramatically increase with each passing year, especially in the United States. Although a wealth of diverse research focused on stimulant addiction has been executed over the past few decades, pharmacological therapies able to successfully treat primary symptoms of stimulant withdrawal symptoms such as anxiety and cravings, or ones that help reduce an addict's risk of relapse, have yet to be clearly identified. Several pharmacological agents have been tested for these specific uses to no avail, including antidepressants, anticonvulsants, and antipsychotics. However, hope remains far from lost, as evidence continues to surface proving that the endocannabinoid system (ECBS) plays a major role in cognitive and physiological activities related to ones present during stimulant addiction. Such activities include the "reward" feeling stemming from stimulant abuse, and responsiveness to stress and drug induced synaptic plasticity, which relates to the power of brain synapses to strengthen or weaken with time as a result of an increase or decrease of activity. The endocannabinoid system's relation to the brain's reward system endows it with strong potential to interfere with, or perhaps even halt, damaging neurological effects seen in those suffering from stimulant addiction.

In relation to relapse, cannabis may lower the risk, as it was also found to affect specific receptors that reduce triggers and temptations which often prompt recovering addicts to fall from sobriety and use again. Similarities in how cannabis and stimulants affect the brain's reward system are unparalleled, pointing to the possible future development of cannabis derived therapies to treat stimulant addiction, due to the fact that the plant is generally well tolerated and non-addictive to the vast majority of the population. Still, further research must be conducted in order for this exciting and seemingly promising therapy to become a readily available treatment option for stimulant addiction, but evidence gathered thus far leaves many hopeful that the unveiling of a ground breaking answer to stimulant abuse may lay on a horizon that is not so distant after all.

Chapter 20

PSYCHOSIS AND SYMPTOMS OF SCHIZOPHRENIA

"They are going to kill me. The people I love are going to kill me."

Those were the thoughts circling through my mind one night as I sat on my bathroom floor in the dark, rocking back and forth, with my head between my knees and the door locked. I could hear my mother, father, and boyfriend outside the door pleading for me to unlock it so they could help me. They sounded genuinely worried. But in my head, I knew better.

Help me? They had no intentions of helping me. The only thing on their agenda was shoving the giant knife they chased me up the stairs with through my heart. My only wish was to drown them out, not to stop going crazy, because in that moment I certainly didn't believe I was going crazy. A person who has been mentally stable for over two decades does not just spontaneously go crazy overnight, or so I thought. I now know the day I found myself in a ball on the bathroom floor hiding from my family, convinced they were vying to murder me, was the first day I experienced a full blown hallucination, one I was entirely wrapped up in and wholeheartedly believed to be real. There was no real knife, and no real threat to my safety.

Approximately a month after the bathroom incident, I went out of town for a week with my boyfriend to meet with a new doctor and have some medical tests done. Apparently on our last night there, I walked straight past my boyfriend and out of our hotel room without saying a word around midnight. When he found me, I was sitting at the end of a hall rocking back and forth with my head between my knees yet again, as I held my legs snugly to my chest and let out muffled cries. He sat down on the floor across from me and attempted to console me, and at first he truly did succeed. Relaxing a bit, I loosened my tense shoulders and rested my back against the wall behind me, giving me a view of the entire hallway. Finally, I could relax. I became convinced I wasn't going crazy, and was merely having an anxiety attack— convinced, until my boyfriend's words faded into the background and I became increasingly distracted by his face as it began to turn upside down. While his head was still on correctly, his facial features were entirely inverted. I tried to conceal the terror I felt, telling myself what I was seeing was not real and would soon end. And it did end, but only in time for terror of a different sort to begin. Behind my boyfriend, an army of life-sized wooden British toy soldiers in black and red uniforms were marching down the hall towards us. I had no choice but to tell him. After all, he had his back turned towards them, pinning him as an easy target for ambush. Turning to assess the British invaders, his demeanor remained calm. The look I expected him to give them, a look of terror and worry, was the one he instead gave me when he turned back around to face me. Instantly, I wondered if he was one of them. Before I could act on my suspicions, though, he picked me up and carried me to our hotel room. As I heard the door to our room click shut behind us, a small glimmer of hope that it was all over with and I was finally safe began to rise within, but its flame was quickly extinguished by the aliens I heard knocking on our door soon after.

As the previous stories briefly detail, I began my descent into a wonderland of nightmarish hallucinations and delusions in a relatively rapid and unexpected manner. Within the course of a month, I was hallucinating on a regular basis. The truth is, clinically speaking; I was insane and belonged in a mental hospital. I was psychotic, paranoid, delusional, and so on. I fit the bill of a mental patient with schizophrenic like tendencies to a "T." The truth also is, in reality, I unknowingly had an out of control case of KPU/HPU (Pyroluria) requiring urgent treatment, lest I desired to descend further down a deceivingly dark spiral of madness. KPU/HPU is a biochemical marker and neurotoxic substance that can be found in the urine of individuals with various illnesses. It has proven to be the underlying cause for many psychiatric conditions, including an estimated 40-70 percent of cases of schizophrenia.

Individuals with Lyme disease and a myriad of other conditions often associated with Lyme disease, including ones with similar methods of ravaging the body, are also susceptible to symptoms of psychosis not unlike those seen in cases of schizophrenia. In fact, to the untrained eye, the behavioral and cognitive patterns exhibited by such individuals are easily mistaken as schizophrenia, leading to many misdiagnoses of schizophrenia and other psychiatric disorders which cause psychosis, are incurable, and require taking medication indefinitely—particularly heavy antipsychotics that change the individual's personality, turning them into somewhat of a zombie who is numb to life, ultimately robbing them of their birth right to feel, as the ability to feel equates with the ability to feel alive, the experience for which we exist. Due to negligence many are stripped of this experience and are misdiagnosed with severe chronic psychiatric conditions that are, in reality, symptoms stemming from underlying treatable conditions such as parasites, nutrient deficiencies, food allergies, or mold or heavy metal toxicities. Illnesses related or similar to Lyme disease that have the potential to manifest symptoms of psychosis and schizophrenic like behavior include babesiosis, ehrlichiosis, mycoplasma pneumonia, toxoplasmosis, stealth virus, borna virus, AIDS, syphilis, CMV, herpes, and strep, to name a few.

Natural treatments potent enough to alleviate symptoms of psychosis and schizophrenia—whether induced by an infectious illness or microbe of some kind, severe nutrient imbalance, or any other origin—are scarce. However, various reports have surfaced claiming cannabis can successfully treat symptoms of psychosis and schizophrenia; but for each of these reports, multiple others have surfaced cautioning of cannabis induced psychosis. While these reports exist on polar opposite ends of the spectrum, the validity of both are well-founded. Cannabis holds the power to either induce or reduce symptoms of psychosis and schizophrenia, as it contains compounds enabling it to do both. The key to treating psychosis and schizophrenia with cannabis lies in identifying the primary compounds in the plant able to alleviate associated symptoms, in order to more adequately identify what strains are best to use.

Cannabis Induced Psychosis

Cannabis has long been linked to psychosis, believed to both induce symptoms of psychosis as well as exacerbate preexisting symptoms of psychosis, most notably those of schizophrenia. Clinical documentation of this belief dates back to 1848, when French psychiatrist Jacques-Joseph Moreau de Tour began studying the effects of cannabis on the brain and body, with his interest particularly fixated on its ability to induce psychosis.[1] To test his theory that it causes psychosis, Moreau used cannabis as an experimental psychotomimetic, a substance which mimics symptoms of psychosis, including but not limited to hallucinations, delusions, and delirium. After observing behavioral changes similar to endogenous psychosis, or psychosis originating from within rather than instigated by external influences, Moreau concluded that THC worked as an excellent experimental psychotomimetic substance, indicating that cannabis strains containing potent amounts of the psychoactive ingredient THC can initiate a symptom picture unparalleled to that of psychosis. Researchers who repeated the study in 2004 using more accurate measurements, scales, and overall means of testing came to the same conclusion as Moreau.[1]

Cannabidiol Reduces Symptoms and Progression of Schizophrenia and Psychotic Conditions by Enhancing Anandamide Signaling

Elevated levels of anandamide, a bioactive lipid that binds to cannabinoid receptors, in cerebrospinal fluid are linked to symptoms of psychosis and schizophrenia. More specifically, they are linked to the prognosis of schizophrenia and psychotic conditions, with the amount to which they are elevated determining the rate at which the psychosis will progress. When exploring anandamide's role in the transitioning of schizophrenic patients from prodromal states of psychosis—the early, initial stages proceeding full blown manifestation of psychotic symptoms— to advanced, final stages of psychosis, researchers measured anandamide levels in the cerebrospinal fluid and serum of subjects in initial prodromal states alongside individuals with good mental health, clinically speaking.[2] On account of ensuring the most accurate results possible, high-performance liquid chromatograph/spectrometry was used for testing.

Schizophrenic patients displayed appreciably higher levels of anandamide compared to test subjects with good mental health. Schizophrenic patients who exhibited anandamide levels that were above average, yet were notably lower in comparison to other patients with schizophrenia and psychosis related conditions, were found to be at greater risk of transitioning from initial prodromal states of psychosis to advanced states of psychosis. This may seem backwards, as elevated levels of anandamide are associated with schizophrenia, a fact which could easily lend to the false assumption that higher levels of anandamide correlate with higher levels of psychosis. On the contrary, the opposite holds true. Anandamidergic upregulation, or enhanced anandamide levels, in the initial prodromal stage of schizophrenia and psychotic conditions are a protective response of the endocannabinoid system activated early on, upon initial onset of symptoms of schizophrenia and psychosis. That the cannabinoid Cannabidiol does not bind to cannabinoid receptors does not render it useless, especially in this case, considering it directly works to inhibit degradation of the endocannabinoid anandamide. Clearly, this is an exciting discovery for those afflicted with schizophrenia and similar conditions, as it offers hope for slower progression of the condition and the possibility of a longer, fuller life.

In a study comparing the effectiveness of cannabidiol and amisulpride, a strong antipsychotic, on schizophrenic symptoms, both medications performed successfully.[3] However, the list of side effects of cannabidiol was significantly less in comparison to that of the prescription antipsychotic amisulpride. Essentially, not only did cannabidiol prove to be an effective treatment for reducing symptoms and progression of schizophrenia by greatly increasing anandamide serum levels, but it did so without simultaneously generating a cascade of undesirable symptoms, as its use is not equipped with a stealthy list of side effects like amisulpride and other prescription drugs are. In short, studies performed using behavioral and neurochemical techniques indicate that the pharmacological profiles of cannabidiol (CBD) and atypical antipsychotic drugs are strikingly similar, making CBD a possible alternative treatment for psychosis. As always, check with your doctor before initiating or changing treatments.

Chapter 21

NAUSEA AND VOMITING

*I*n the next chapter we discuss cachexia, or "wasting syndrome," a phenomenon seen in individuals with certain chronic illnesses that causes severe malnutrition. If not addressed, highly dangerous repercussions may occur. Nausea and vomiting are dangerous for the same reason as cachexia—if allowed to continue for too long without successful intervention, severe malnutrition may ensue. Fortunately, it appears cannabis may be of help. Its anti-emetic, or anti-nausea, effects have been studied more than any of its other medicinal benefits, and are one of the primary reasons why doctors prescribe it to patients.

GW Pharmaceuticals compiled data of 768 patients from results of state-sponsored studies on the effects of cannabis on chemo-therapy-induced nausea and vomiting. Approximately 76-88 percent of the 768 patients reported relief from nausea and vomiting following oral administration of THC (i.e. oils), while 70-100 percent of patients reported relief from nausea and vomiting after smoking cannabis. The majority of other medical studies on cannabis tend to favor oral consumption, primarily oils, as opposed to smoking, claiming it a healthier option. However, smoking often proves advantageous when attempting to control nausea and vomiting, due to the risk of further provoking symptoms by consuming the herb orally when the body is already struggling to hold food and liquids down.

Delta-8-THC Prevents Nausea

A study found delta-8-tetrahydrocannabinol (delta-8-THC), a compound in cannabis similar to actual THC (delta-9-tetrahydrocannabinol) but less potent, effectively treats nausea. The study was conducted on children undergoing chemotherapy treatments for cancer, making its results all the more remarkable, as controlling nausea in children undergoing chemotherapy is typically a significantly more difficult task than it is in adults. Delta-8-THC completely prevented nausea and vomiting in children when taken two hours before chemotherapy treatments.

Anti-nausea Effects of CBD

CBD suppresses nausea and vomiting by inhibiting 5-HT3 receptors, similar to prescription 5-HT3 receptor agonist medications used to treat nausea and vomiting, such as the widely prescribed anti-nausea drug Ondansetron. When serotonin is released in the small intestine, it stimulates vagal afferent nerves by interacting with 5-HT3 receptors, which provokes the vomiting reflex. 5-HT3 receptor agonists block the vomiting reflex by preventing serotonin from binding to 5-HT3 receptors in the small intestine and the solitary tract nucleus (STN) and chemoreceptor trigger zone (CTZ) sites of the central nervous system.

Chapter 22

CACHEXIA OR "WASTING SYNDROME"

For many people, mostly women, who I have met who have Lyme disease and/or related infections, an unhealthy amount of weight gain and an almost absolute inability to lose weight are among their most prominent symptoms. In fact, at least half of the women I know with Lyme disease and/or associated infections find this seemingly unwarranted weight gain that they are unable to shake to be one of their most bothersome symptoms, primarily on physical self-acceptance, self-esteem, and social levels. On the opposite end of the totem pole are those with Lyme disease and Lyme disease co-infections who lose a significant amount of weight without actively trying to, and are then unable to gain any weight, regardless of their activities. Having lost 20 pounds upon the onset of chronic Lyme disease symptoms, and miserably failing to gain (much less consistently keep) more than a single one of my stolen pounds back over the course of the two years following their hijacking, it suffices to say

I am one such individual accounting for the population making up this end of the spectrum.

When I lost 20 pounds within a month of moving into a mold infested condo, beckoning previously dormant spirochetes and bacteria to life, I thought little of it. I had 30 other problematic symptoms to worry about during that time period, on a good day—must I mention, I was in hypochondriac mode? When I began to catch on that I was different from many other women with Lyme disease, as they struggled with obesity while my light weight remained unwavering, I didn't really catch on to anything useful, but rather a vain mind made illusion. I fancied myself lucky, not having to stress over what I looked like, knowing I could throw on anything without looking fat. I doted on the idea that my body was naturally petite, allowing me to wear size zero and sometimes double zero jeans from middle school—except, my petite figure was certainly not natural, nor was the way size zero and double zero jeans fit it snugly yet comfortably like an immaculately designed custom made glove. All of this, and I still did not feel there was anything wrong with my initial, significant weight loss followed by an absolute inability to gain weight. Admittedly, I saw it as somewhat of a blessing, until the day I realized my feet had shrunk an entire shoe size shook me free of my delusion. Having been a size eight for a good chunk of my life, I was dumbfounded when my shoes that had been slightly slipping off at times since I fell ill eventually began doing so at all times. Eventually, not a single pair of my size eight shoes properly fit me, forcing me to purchase size seven replacements. At that point, logic finally showed up to the equation and I realized a person does not just shrink an entire shoe size. Perhaps, if one was overweight and lost a significant amount of weight their shoes would then fit loosely, but even this scenario didn't apply to me. Like a tidal wave, the words "I'm wasting away" flooded through me, and it turned out they were quite an eerily appropriate choice of words. As I soon learned, my loss of fat and bone mass were attributed to cachexia, or "wasting syndrome," from Mycoplasma—infectious bacteria that scavenge nutrients and cause severe malnutrition in their hosts.

Cachexia, or "wasting syndrome," is a complex metabolic syndrome that causes a loss in appetite, dramatic weight loss and muscle atrophy in individuals who are not actively dieting or intentionally attempting to lose weight. The syndrome, which also causes fatigue and weakness, is characterized by wasting of adipose tissue and skeletal muscle. Cachexia is prominent in advanced infections of mycoplasma, as well as in various other chronic diseases and conditions, including but not limited to Multiple Sclerosis, Type 1 Diabetes, HIV and cancer. Scientists have yet to identify the exact mechanism(s) responsible for manifesting symptoms of cachexia and, without a direct bodily process to target, developing drugs to adequately treat the syndrome is an undeniably complex and challenging process. Drugs to treat cachexia do exist, and more are in development, but success rates of such drugs are less than impressive. So, the idea that the drugs in development for cachexia will be able to treat cachexia on a mass scale, across a broad spectrum of conditions that cause it, is not extremely promising. Of course, the only way to properly treat the syndrome may be to treat the underlying cause, such as mycoplasma and/or any other illnesses responsible for its onset. Even if this is the case, therapies alternative to currently available unsuccessful conventional ones that are able to at least reduce symptoms of cachexia to some degree throughout the course of treatment are certainly worth pursuing.

Using Cannabis as an Appetite Stimulant

As an appetite stimulant, cannabis may reduce symptoms, inhibit progression, and improve prognosis of cachexia by reversing weight loss, and inhibiting tissue deterioration and muscle wasting from decreased nutritional intake from the increased metabolic demand chronic illnesses place on the body. Malnutrition from illnesses such as Mycoplasma, which causes a wealth of nutritional deficiencies, have potentially devastating consequences, with the worst being nothing short of death itself.

Cannabis promotes appetite stimulation by interacting with the endocannabinoid system. Cannabinoids, namely THC, bind to cannabinoid receptors involved in appetite regulation. THC also interacts with the leptin pathway in the endocannabinoid system, which ultimately plays a critical role in appetite stimulation by managing leptin signaling—the bodily process responsible for maintaining healthy levels of leptin, the primary hormone the hypothalamus uses to assess the body's nutritional state and moderate food intake.

A standard means of treating wasting from cachexia on a broad scale is as dire as it is elusive. While drugs for treating cachexia exist, many are almost entirely ineffective. Some drugs work well for treating cachexia caused by a select condition, but are contraindicated in those with cachexia caused by other conditions. Progestogens are a perfect example. Currently, progestogens are the best available treatment option for cancer induced cachexia but are not recommended for use in individuals with cachexia from Lyme disease and Lyme disease co-infections, as they are a class of steroid hormones and steroids hold potential to markedly worsen the severity of these infections. With an increase in appetite as one of its most well-known side effects, cannabis may be a more advantageous option than synthetic drugs for treating cachexia on a wide scale, among several different ill-nesses. Because of this and numerous other medicinal benefits of cannabis mentioned herein, not to mention numerous other ones not even included in this book, cannabis is a golden con-tender for treating and/or managing symptoms of Lyme disease, Lyme disease co-infections, and related conditions for many.

Chapter 23

FINAL CONCLUSIONS ABOUT CANNABIS, THE INTELLIGENCE OF PLANTS, AND BACTERIA'S ELUSIVE ROLE IN EVOLUTION

*"Plants are living entities and what you do when you heal with plant medicine is that you bring together the living entity of a plant, with the living entity of the person, with the living entity of the organ system through the introductory medium of the herbalist. Your perception has to be sensitive enough to understand how to do that and to perceive what happens inside the person when they are all introduced. Different herbs may affect the body similarly but they often affect the psychological structure very differently. The only way to know how they affect people psychologically as well as physically is to **have a personal relationship with the plant.**"*

-Julie McIntyre, Herbalist and Author of
SEX AND THE INTELLIGENCE OF THE HEART:
NATURE, INTIMACY AND SEXUAL ENERGY

I used to ignorantly mock those who spoke of conversing with plants and actually talking with them, not just to them, much less forming strong relationships with them. I would scoff at the very idea, thinking such people must be smoking a certain kind of plant if it talks to them—cannabis, to be specific. After all, I admittedly felt ignorantly strong about the lack of necessity for the use of cannabis, as I was conditioned to believe it was nothing more than a "harmful drug" growing up. Medicinally speaking, I knew close to nothing about the herb, the herb that would in turn forgive my foolish mockery in an instant to save my life.

Ironically, I was not the slightest bit high when a plant spoke to me for the first time. Also, ironically, it was the soothing touch of cannabis itself, beckoning me at 3:00 A.M. in my own dark night of the soul; as I lingered on the brink of life and death, struggling to decide whether or not it was worth the effort to summon the courage and strength to take my next breath, and then the next and the next, or if I should just give up and die. I saw a bag of largely ignored cannabis next to my bed, the one I touched as if it were tainted, using it only to control my seizures and, to my surprise, it spoke to me. Not by words. I am not sure it is accurate to say by feeling, either. Rather, the message was delivered through the gentle touch of a deep sense of knowing. The kind that digs deeper than thoughts, than words, than the vocal system, and certainly deeper than any of the preconceived notions we are all conditioned to believe about the world from a young age. Intuition. In inviting me to rest my weary life in its hands, after years of betrayal from everyone and everything I knew, an herb offered me a vessel to once again place my trust without fear of being hurt, of being judged, of being harmed.

An ancient truth murmured among our indigenous ancestors many moons ago, one still sifting through hearts of a few present day people with an insatiable hunger for the purest form of love attainable, is that of knowing what it is to live with nature rather than on nature at a level so deep that no words exist to describe it to those who have not yet journeyed there. This sacred truth sits at the core of full healing, the place where mind, body, and spirit gracefully shift into alignment. It proclaims one must have no doubt in the plant they are using to heal themselves. In fact, they should not be merely using the plant at all, but working with it, respecting it, and above all offering it sincere gratitude. One must wholeheartedly trust in their chosen plant's ability to heal them. The relationship between the healer and the healing, or the plant and the patient, must be faithful, built on trust, and free of fear.

Paradoxically, I had never fully trusted in any other herb, beyond a shadow of doubt, to heal me, regardless of research and first-hand accounts of their impressive abilities to heal Lyme disease and Lyme disease co-infections. In hindsight, it seems insane that the previous herbs in which I did not trust had been used by many people, including ones I personally knew, to treat Lyme disease; while on the other hand, the herb I knew relatively nothing about, and had not heard of a single other person with Lyme disease utilizing for medicinal purposes, was the one I placed my full trust in for the first time in two years without a trace of hesitation. I guess that's just it, though, the only soul I truly needed to know was my own, as the ability to truly know anyone or anything must always start at the still place within each of us. And so, in the most unexpected of ways in the darkness of the most unexpected of nights, my soul involuntarily shifted into the source of stillness and serenity within all beings, prompting me to release my grasp on the knife I was holding with its blade to my left wrist, to instead grasp for the herb whose ability to heal me was something I knew close to nothing about. In the dead of the night, I dismissed my grip on suicide and instinctively held tight to my new shot at true happiness, my new shot at life; and thus began my journey to once again discovering what it is like to know more than the physical sensation of breathing, and instead know the invisible deep feeling of all that surrounds each inhale and exhale, my heart pounding with overwhelming gratitude beneath, leaving no room for worries about death, as I became filled to my fingertips with the ecstasy of a long forgotten freedom—the feeling of being alive.

While the human race strives to create synthetic drugs for drug resistant bacteria like MRSA, plants, specifically cannabis in regards to MRSA, have proven to successfully treat these infections. What we fail miserably to see is that it is not plants alone that were endowed with this gift, but us too, as such a gift is readily available to save us in many areas which man made drugs are failing to treat. The gift was always meant to be shared with us, we were always and will always be meant to coexist with nature, whether we deny the call to indulge in a relationship with it or not.

The fact that a life changing, and often times lifesaving, plant like cannabis is the subject pitted in the middle of a boiling nationwide controversy means that, in reality, at the root of it all, the hysteria may not actually be about cannabis at all. Perhaps, a large part stems from an unspoken truth (as many are unconscious of it, even while partaking), a war among the egos. In the midst of the "war on cannabis," the herb remains untainted, with relatively small amounts of people reaping its lifesaving benefits in comparison to all of the people afflicted with life threatening or disabling illnesses who could be saved, but sit idly by. After all, that is what much of society has done—sat idly by while sick individuals are denied natural medications capable of putting an end to their suffering. Rather than placing focus on the good cannabis can do, focus is placed on the (what many believe to be) bad things people have done with it. At some point, we must stop debating for the sake of hearing our own voices and sit and consider the possibility that society has a much larger problem on its hands than the legalization of cannabis if a "brainless plant" can so easily provoke mass conflict among humans by simply being. Perhaps, it is because something without a "brain" is taking over ours, or, perhaps it is because these plants really are intelligent, and we are wasting our time fighting because we have so much to learn from them. And this brings us to the regrettably, shamefully often overlooked intelligence of plants.

The Intelligence of Plants

The idea that plants possess intelligence worthy of in depth exploration is an idea still largely scoffed at, despite the emergence of research suggesting otherwise. In large part, this is due to the widespread belief that "intelligence" and "brains" are inextricably connected, that the two must coexist to exist at all. The problem with this is our perception of what a "brain" is. When defining the brain, we fixate too much on the physicals, like that it exists strictly within a skull; and not enough on the invisibles, such as how it functions. When looking deeper into the characteristics of plants, though, we begin to find they have impressively elegant mechanisms, ones typically reserved only for those with brains.

Plants communicate chemically, in a manner which we cannot directly decipher. For example, an insect attack is stimulated and the release of volatile chemicals is instigated when sagebrush leaves are clipped in the spring, resulting in a significant reduction of the extent to which both the clipped plant and the unclipped plants around it suffer. Chemical communication amongst plants may also be of benefit to farmers, as research by a chemical ecologist at the University of Missouri revealed the following: plant-distress chemicals may be used to prime plant defenses, thus eliminating the need for pesticides.[1] Plants also display excellent hearing capabilities, a fact well demonstrated in a study showing how in reaction to the sound of a caterpillar munching on a leaf, plants secrete defensive chemicals as a response to a perceived potential threat from a foreign sound.[2]

Although plants do not have "brains," in the sense which us humans define them—meaning they consist within the boundaries of a skull—, they possess intricate neuronal networks with more neurons than the human brain. One might say their roots are their brains, and since they are not confined by a skull like the human brain, they are able to expand infinitely, with no existing limit on the knowledge which they obtain. Plants learn, remember, react, and sense in ways similar to humans. In fact, sensory abilities of plants are so distinguished and immaculate that they are able to gather all sensory data from one day, and integrate it to formulate an appropriate response.

Plants not only produce anesthetics, they respond to them as well. This does not, however, directly prove plants feel pain—a topic still up for debate among scientists. What is clear is that plants possess all of the same senses attributed to humans, a fact surprising to some; as well as ones which do not fall under the category of human senses, a fact surprising to most. Aside from their abilities to feel, hear, and taste, plants sense obstacles able to impede the growth of their roots before coming into contact with them, and shift their direction of growth accordingly. They are also able to sense gravity and the presence of water. Exactly how plants have the same senses as humans, not to mention in some ways more distinguished ones, all while void of what we envision a brain to be, remains a mystery, its answers lying in the vastly unexplored terrain of plant consciousness and intelligence. What we know for sure is that, like us, plants produce neurotransmitters such as dopamine, serotonin, and other chemicals to send and receive electrical signals. To a large degree, concrete details beyond this remain a mystery—one that some scientists are working to unveil. Other, less humble ones, of course, label the very idea of plant consciousness and intelligence as quackery, still unaware that true science often lies in the beauty of not knowing.

Bacteria's Elusive Role in Evolution

I refer to bacteria's role in evolution as "elusive" not because their mechanisms are truly sneaky, but because humans are, to a large degree, entirely oblivious of their importance in evolution. In fact, the earth's very existence is dependent on the existence of bacteria. As Stephen Buhner so eloquently put it, "If humans disappear from the earth, the earth will be fine. If bacteria disappear, all life will cease to exist. There are organisms here far more intelligent than human beings. We've been taught our brain structure is the most sophisticated on the planet—it's not. There are organisms here that have brain neurons that far exceed our own order by 10 ...100 ...1,000 times."[3] We are composed of bacteria. If we killed all the bacteria inside of us, we would also kill ourselves and die almost immediately.

Both good bacteria and bacteria harmful to our health exist. Still, in an evolutionary sense, it is debatable that bacteria harmful to our health are "bad" bacteria, so I refrain from labeling them as so. Perhaps they do not want to destroy us, but to morph and evolve into new organisms, just like they have done since the beginning of not only their lives on earth, but far before the beginning of human life. Existing at least 3 ½ billion years, bacteria hold the title of the oldest life form on the entire planet.[3]

Few would argue that the number of different types of bacterial infections in general are steadily on the rise, much less ones with such intriguingly complex defense mechanisms that, even when a drug or treatment of some sort that can kill them IS developed, they quickly turn its weaknesses into their strengths and rapidly evolve to evade the threat. Yes, we are constantly trying to create new ways to successfully fight the bacteria threatening our lives, but the bacteria are also creating new ways to successfully fight the weapons threatening their lives—not us, but the medications we are using to wage war. Do you understand what I am saying? Bacteria in those with potentially fatal diseases, such as Lyme disease, do not actually want to kill US. If we die, they die, and they do not want to die. They want to survive, meaning we, their hosts, must also stay alive. We have never considered the issue that bacteria harmful to our health might be bigger than us, that it might be an ecological message. We have long thought the goal of bacteria with potential to harm our health, such as spirochetes, is to kill us. Perhaps they have a much greater agenda though, a collective goal, not unlike the one that is the very reason we are alive today—evolution.

In believing ourselves superior to nature, placing ourselves above all other life forms and living in a way in which we live on the earth rather than with the earth, we have voluntarily made ourselves inferior to other species in regards to the rate at which we are evolving. Humans have destroyed, and continue to destroy, the natural environment. Bacteria such as Borrelia spirochetes are altering their mechanisms quite quickly in response, and humans are beginning to feel the impact more and more with each passing day. The more we destroy the environment, the more disease we face. As we continue to damage the ecosystem, bacteria like Lyme spirochetes continue to respond by quickly altering their structure to ensure their survival, and we are starting to feel the repercussions on a grand scale. Reducing forest and wilderness areas has also reduced the number of mammals, birds, and other nonhuman hosts available for ticks and other vectors to latch onto and infect with illnesses like Lyme disease.

Evolution is actively occurring whether we want it to or not. We have no say in the matter. We do, however, have a say in the nature in which it does so to some degree, in whether or not involvement of the human species contributes to it productively or destructively. Bacteria are rapidly evolving, and we would be wise to follow suit, to get to know the inner workings of bacteria like Lyme spirochetes coursing through our blood deeply and intimately. Then, rather than taking that knowledge through the doors of a lab to create pharmaceuticals to undermine the bacteria, perhaps we should walk out our doors and into the wildness of nature's pharmacy where plants like cannabis that are capable of healing us exist, ready and willing to forge relationships with us, waiting to show us that unlike man made pharmaceutical drugs, they can heal us without simultaneously harming us too. It is illogical and debatably useless to try and resolve one health problem in a way that at the same time generates new ones, much like we see in the case of long term antibiotic use for example.

Emergence of drug resistant bacteria is on the rise, and coming with it is an emergence in awareness that plant medicine is not only helpful but is essential to our survival. Although, collectively, the rate at which we are waking up to this fact unfortunately remains quite slow. Eventually, though, the one inevitable truth determining the fate of the human race will grow glaringly unavoidable: living in a manner in which man lives with the land, as opposed to merely on it—suppressing his inherent greed for power over other life forms to pay heed to his evolutionary need to live harmoniously with them—is not simply a way of life. Ultimately, it is the only way to life.

Acknowledgements

Further thanks goes out to my publisher, Bryan Rosner, whose gentle approach to working with me made the process of writing my first book seem like heaven in comparison to the horror stories I have heard about publishers from other writers.

I hold an immense amount of gratitude for Julie McIntyre, whose work made my healing process much more harmonious; and although she does not know it, for reinstating my wavering courage half-way through the writing of this book by informing me that speaking with excruciating honesty is the highest form of human compassion -contrary to what society had previously taught me, yet nonetheless deeply true.

Chris, for walking through the fog of lost time with me, for teaching me that just because I believe something to be true does not mean it is, for continuously prying open the closed parts of my mind, and for showing me that even on my worst days there is always something new I can learn and become better at ...and most importantly, for the time I called and said I felt I was a burden to my friends and family because I had Lyme disease, and he said, "if you must be a burden, at least be worthy of being one." Those words changed everything for me.

And Seth, for offering me insight on cannabis throughout the process of writing this book, and for repeatedly enduring my frantic writing fits during the middle of various nights; and above all, thanks for being a partner who endlessly loves me, supports me, and inspires me.

References

CHAPTER 1: CANNABIS AS A BACTERICIDAL AND FOR SYMPTOM PICTURE REDUCTION

Cited references:

1. World Health Organization. (2014, April 30). *WHO's first global report on antibiotic resistance reveals serious, worldwide threat to public health.* Retrieved November 13, 2014, from http://www.who.int/mediacentre/news/releases/2014/amr-report/en/

2. Ericson, J. (2013, July 30). *Marijuana Kills MRSA and Inhibits Prions That Cause Neurodegenerative Disease; Still Recognized by Feds As a Dangerous Drug.* Retrieved November 13, 2014, from http://www.medicaldaily.

com/marijuana-kills-mrsa-and-inhibits-prions-cause-neurodegenerative-disease-still-recognized-feds

3. Appendino, G., Gibbons, S., Gianna, A. et. al. (2008). Antibacterial Cannabinoids from Cannabis sativa: A Structure—Active Study. Journal of Natural Products, 71: 1427-1430. Print.

Other references for this chapter:

*   Wright, P.M., Seiple, I.B., & Myers, A.G. (2014). The Evolving Role of Chemical Synthesis in Antibacterial Drug Discovery. *Angew Chem Int Ed, 53*(34), 8840-8869.

*   Russo, E. B. (2001). "Taming THC: potential cannabis synergy and phytocannabinoid-terpenoid entourage effects." *British Journal of Pharmacology, 163*(7): 1344–1364.

*   Dorm, D. (2013, September 23). Terpenes May Improve Effectiveness Of Medical Marijuana. Retrieved from http://www.medicaljane.com/2013/09/23/terpenes-may-improve-effectiveness-of-medical-marijuana/

CHAPTER 2: CHEMICAL CONSTITUENTS OF CANNABIS

Cited references:

1. Russo, E. (2006). Cannabis and Cannabis Extracts: Greater Than the Sum of Their Parts? In Handbook of cannabis therapeutics: From bench to bedside (pp. 103-132). New York: Haworth Press.

2. Brenneisen, R. (2007). Chemistry and Analysis of Phytocannabinoids and Other Cannabis Constituents. In M. ElSohly (Ed.), Marijuana and the cannabinoids (pp. 17-49). Totowa, N.J.: Humana Press.

3. Komori, T., Fujiwara, R., Tanida, M., Normura, J., and Yokoyama, M.M. (1996). Effects of citrus fragrance on immune function and depressive states. *Neuroimmunonod.* 2(3): 174-80

4. Gwanzura, L., McFarland, W., Alexander, D., Burke, R.L., & Katzenstein, D. (1998). Association between human immunodeficiency virus and herpes simplex virus type 2 seropositivity among male factory workers in Zimbabwe. *J Infect Dis.* 177(2):481-4

5. Long, X., Fan, M., Bigsby, R., & Nephew, K. (2008). Apigenin Inhibits Antiestrogen-resistant Breast Cancer Cell Growth through Estrogen Receptor-α-dependent and -independent Mechanisms. Mol Cancer Ther., 7(7), 2096-2108.

Other references for this chapter:

- *The Therapeutic Uses of Cannabis and Cannabinoids.* (n.d.). Retrieved September 18, 2014, from http://www.unitedpatientsgroup.com/resources/how-medical-marijuana-works

- Buhner, S. (2005). *Healing Lyme: Natural prevention and treatment of Lyme borreliosis and its coinfections.* Randolph, Vt.: Raven Press.

- Handcrafted Whole Plant Extracted Cannabis and Hemp Based Medicine, M. (n.d.). The Spectrum of the Cannabis Plant. Retrieved September 16, 2014.

- D'Souza, R., & Dhume, V. (1991, April 1). Gastric cytoprotection. *Indian J Physiol Pharmaco.* 35(2): 88-9. Retrieved pn September 20, 2014 from http://www.ncbi.nlm.nih.gov/pubmed/1791051

- Boubaker, J., Mansour, H.B., Ghedira, K., Chekir-Ghediral, L. (2011). Antimutagenic and free radical scavenger effects of leaf extracts from Accacia salicina.*Annals of Clinical Microbiology and Antimicrobials.* 10(37). doi:10.1186/1476-0711-10-37

- McPartland, J.M. (1997). Cannabis as a repellent crop and botanical pesticide. *J Internat Hemp Assoc* 4(2):89-94

- Buhler, D.R., & Miranda, C. (2000, November). Antioxidant Activities of Flavonoids. Retrieved September 25, 2014, from http://lpi.oregonstate.edu/f-w00/flavonoid.html

- Musonda, C.A., & Chipman, J.K. (1998). Quercetin inhibits hydrogen peroxide induced NF-kB DNA binding activity and DNA damage in HepG2 cells. Carcinogen (19): 1583-9.

CHAPTER 3: STRAINS AND SPECIES OF CANNABIS

- Yablan, J.S. (2007, February 27). *What Are the Differences between Cannabis Indica and Cannabis Sativa, and How Do They Vary in Their Potential Medical Utility?* Retrieved from http://medicalmarijuana.procon.org/view.answers.php?questionID=000638

- Patients Marijuana Caregiver Services. (2011). Cannabis Sativa vs. Cannabis Indica and Hybrid Strains. Retrieved from http://www.patientsmarijuana.org/index.html

CHAPTER 4: FORMS AND METHODS OF CANNABIS USE

Cited references:

1. Sidney, S. The British Medical Journal, Sept. 20, 2003; vol 327: pp 635-636.

Other references for this chapter:

- Paula, E., & Media, D. (n.d.). Nutrients That Yield Food Energy. Retrieved September 29, 2014, from http://healthyeating.sfgate.com/nutrients-yield-food-energy-7724.html

- The Great Wide World of Cannabis Concentrates. (n.d.). Retrieved September 29, 2014, from http://www.leafly.com/knowledge-center/cannabis-101/the-great-wide-world-of-cannabis-concentrates

- Colorado Pot Guide. (2014, February 6). Different types of marijuana concentrates available in Colorado. Retrieved September 29, 2014, from https://www.coloradopotguide.com/colorado-marijuana-blog/2014/february/06/different-types-of-marijuana-concentrates-available-in-colorado/

- UnitedPatientsGroup (2014, February 13) Cannabis Infused Coconut Oil—How to and the benefits! (n.d.). Retrieved September 29, 2014, from http://www.unitedpatientsgroup.com/blog/2014/02/23/cannabis-infused-coconut-oil-how-to-and-the-benefits/

- Campbell, G. (2012)*Pot, Inc. Inside Medical Marijuana, America's Most Outlaw Industry* New York, NY: Sterling Publishing

- Americans for Safe Access. (2011, February 1). Chronic Pain and Medical Cannabis. Retrieved September 25, 2014, from http://www.denverrelief.com/blog/wp-content/uploads/2011/06/pain_brochure.pdf

CHAPTER 5: SAFETY OF CANNABIS USE

Cited references:

1. Americans for Safe Access. (2014, January 1). *Information on Cannabis Safety.* Retrieved October 2, 2014, from http:// www.safeaccessnow.org/cannabis_safety

2. Dreher, M.C., Nugent, K., & Hudgins, R. (1994). Prenatal Marijuana Exposure and Neonatal Outcomes in Jamaica: An Ethnographic Study. *Pediatrics, 93*(2), 254-260.

3. DeLisi, L.E., Bertisch, H.C., & Szulc, K.U. (2006). A Preliminary DTI study showing no brain structural change associated with adolescent cannabis use. Harm Reduction Journal,3(17).

Other references for this chapter:

• The Natural Standard Research Collaboration. (2013, November 1). *Marijuana (Cannabis sativa): Safety.* Retrieved October 2, 2014, from http://www.mayoclinic.org/ drugs-supplements/marijuana/safety/hrb-20059701

• Truthonpot.com. (2013, July 6). *Pesticides, Bacteria And Mold In Cannabis: The Risks.* Retrieved October 2, 2014, from http://www.truthonpot.com/2013/07/06/ pesticides-bacteria-and-mold-in-cannabis-the-risks/

• Feature, S. (2014, February 25). *The Health Risks of Smoking Marijuana.* Retrieved October 2, 2014, from http://www.webmd.com/news/breaking-news/ marijuana-on-main-street/is-marijuana-safe-web

- Brady, P. (1999, January 1). Ganja mothers, ganja babies | Cannabis Culture. Retrieved October 1, 2014, from http://www.cannabisculture.com/articles/1422.html

CHAPTER 6: LEGALITIES

- Campbell, G. (2012). *Pot, Inc.: Inside medical marijuana, America's most outlaw industry*. New York: Sterling.

- Governing.com. (n.d.). *State Marijuana Laws Map.* Retrieved October 1, 2014, from http://www.governing.com/gov-data/state-marijuana-laws-map-medical-recreational.html

- Chapter seven

- NORML. (n.d.). NORML.org—Working to Reform Marijuana Laws. Retrieved October 1, 2014, from http://norml.org/laws/

CHAPTER 7: JOINT PAIN

Cited references:

1. Fitzcharles, M. et. al. (2012). "Clinical implications for cannabinoid use in the rheumatic diseases: Potential for help or harm?". *Arthritis & Rheumatism,* 64: 2417–2425. Print.

2. Griffing, G.T. (2013, September 12). Endocannabinoids. Retrieved from http://emedicine.medscape.com/ article/1361971-overview#aw2aab6b3

CHAPTER 8: NERVE PAIN

Cited references:

1. Science, Leaf (2014, April 21). *Cannabis May Be Best Treatment For Fibromyalgia, Survey Finds.* Retrieved from http://www.leafscience.com/2014/04/21/ cannabis-best—   treatment-fibromyalgia/

2. Armentano, P. (2013, January 3). Study: Vaporized, Low-Potency Cannabis Reduces Problematic Nerve Pain. Retrieved from http://www.alternet.org/study-vaporized-low-potency-cannabis-reduces-problematic-nerve-pain

Other references for this chapter:

• Jimena, F., et al. (2011). "Cannabis Use in Patients with Fibromyalgia: Effect on Symptoms Relief and Health-Related Quality of Life". *PLoS One: A Peer-Reviewed, Open Access Journal.* 6(4): e18440. doi: 10.1371/journal. pone.0018440

• Wilsey, B., et. Al. (2012). "Low Dose Vaporized Cannabis Significantly Improves Neuropathic Pain." The Journal of Pain, 14(2); 136-148. doi: 10.1016/j.pain.2012.10.009

CHAPTER 9: MIGRAINES

Cited references:

1. Wenk, G.L. (2013 September 16). *Marijuana for Migraines: Migraine Sufferers have few options for reducing their headache pain.* Retrieved from http://www.psychologytoday.com/blog/your-brain-food/201309/marijuana-migraines

2. Russon, E. (2001). Hemp for Headache: An In-Depth Historical and Scientific Review of Cannabis in Migraine Treatment. Journal of Cannabis Therapeutics, 1(2).

CHAPTER 10: MUSCLE SPASTICITY

Cited references:

1. Mack, A., & Joy, J. (2001). Marijuana and Muscle Spasticity. In *Marijuana as Medicine? The Science Beyond the Controversy* (pp.105-114). Washington, D.C.: National Academy Press

2. Vaney, C., Heinzel-Gutenbrunner, M., Jobin, P., Tschopp, F., Gattlen, B., Hagen, U., ... Reif, M. (2004). Efficacy, Safety And Tolerability Of An Orally Administered Cannabis Extract In The Treatment Of Spasticity In Patients With Multiple Sclerosis: A Randomized, Double-blind, Placebo-controlled, Crossover Study. Multiple Sclerosis, 417-424.

CHAPTER 11: BRAIN INFLAMMATION AND MEMORY LOSS

Cited references:

1. Alleyene, R. (2008, November 19). *Marijuana may improve memory and help fight Alzheimer's.* Retrieved October 2, 2014, from http://www.telegraph.co.uk/science/science-news/3485163/Marijuana-may-improve-memory-and-help-fight-Alzheimers.html

2. Wenk, PhD, G. (2010, July 14). Maintaining Memories with Marijuana. Retrieved September 13, 2014, from http://www.psychologytoday.com/blog/your-brain-food/201007/maintaining-memories-marijuana

Other references for this chapter:

• MedlinePlus, U.S. National Library of Medicine. (2013, September 8). *Encephalitis.* Retrieved from http://nlm.nih.gov/medlineplus/ency/article/001415

• White, S. (2013, September 21). *Marijuana May Prevent Memory Loss by Reducing Brain Inflammation.* Retrieved October 2, 2014, from http://www.collective-evolution.com/2013/09/21/marijuana-may-prevent-memory-loss-by-reducing-brain-inflammation/

• Keim, B. (2008, November 19). Marijuana Could Be Good for Memory—But Not if You Get High | WIRED. Retrieved September 2, 2014, from http://www.wired.com/2008/11/marijuana-could/

CHAPTER 12: SLEEP DISORDERS

Cited References

1. Reinarman, C., Nunberg, H., Lanthier, F., & Heddleston, T. (2011). Who Are Medical Marijuana Patients? Population Characteristics from Nine California Assessment Clinics. *Journal of Psychoactive Drugs, 43*(2), 128-135.

2. Ware, M., Doyle, C., Woods, R., Lynch, M., & Clark, A. (2003). Cannabis Use For Chronic Non-cancer Pain: Results Of A Prospective Survey. *Pain, 102*(1), 211-216.

3. Murillo-Rodriguez, E., Poot-Ake, A., Arias-Carrion, O., Pacheco-Pantoja, E., Fuente-Ortegon, A., & Arankowsky-Sandoval, G. (2011). The Emerging Role of the Endocannabinoid System in the Sleep-Wake Cycle Modulation. *Central Nervous System Agents in Medicinal Chemistry,11*(3), 189-196.

4. Prasad, B., Radulovacki, M., & Carley, D. (2013). Proof of Concept Trial of Dronabinol in Obstructive Sleep Apnea. Frontiers in Psychiatry, 4(1). Retrieved November 27, 2014, from doi: 10.3389/fpsyt.2012.00001

Other references for this chapter:

*   LeafScience. (2014, June 3). *Marijuana And Sleep: What's The Connection?*—Leaf Science. Retrieved September 11, 2014, from http://www.leafscience.com/2014/06/03/marijuana-sleep-whats-connection/

- Cousens, K., & DiMascio, A. (1973). (−)δ9 THC as an hypnotic. *Psychopharmacologia, 33*(4), 355-364.

- Clark, A., Ware, M., Yazer, E., Murray, T., & Lynch, M. (2004). Patterns of cannabis use among patients with multiple sclerosis. *Neurology, 62*(11), 2098-2100.

- Truthonpot.com. (2012, November 12). Marijuana and Sleep: The Facts. Retrieved October 8, 2014, from http://www.truthonpot.com/2012/11/03/marijuana-and-sleep/

- Ware MA, Fitzcharles MA, Joseph L, Shir Y (2010) The effects of nabilone on sleep in fibromyalgia: results of a randomized controlled trial. Anesth Analg 110: 604–610.

- Fiz, J., Durán, M., Capellà, D., Carbonell, J., Farré, M., & García, A. (2011). Cannabis Use in Patients with Fibromyalgia: Effect on Symptoms Relief and Health-Related Quality of Life.*PLoS ONE, 6*(4), E18440-E18440.

- Lashley, F. (2003). A Review of Sleep in Selected Immune and Autoimmune Disorders.Holistic Nursing Practice, 17(2), 65-80.

CHAPTER 13: PTSD AND MENTAL TRAUMA

Cited References

1. Bransfield, R.C. (2008). Posttraumatic Stress Disorder and Infectious Encephalopathies. *Lyme Disease Alliance Newsletter.* Retrieved from http://www.mentalhealthandillness.com/Articles/PosttraumaticStressDisorder.Html

2. Mechoulam, R. (2010). General Use of Cannabis for PTSD Symptoms. Retrieved from http://www.veteransformedicalmarijuana.org/content/general-use-cannabis-ptsd-symptoms

Other references for this chapter:

- Neumeister, A., Norandin, M.D., Pietrzak, R.H., et al.(2013). "Elevated brain CB1 receptor availability in post-traumatic stress disorder: a positron emission tomography study." *Molecular Psychiatry.* 18, 1034-1040. doi: 10.1038/mp.2013.61

- Buhner, S.H. (2013, May). Lyme Disease: Some Thoughts On Its Co-infections. *Wisdom Magazine.* Retrieved from http://www.wisdom-magazine.com/article.aspx/3130

- Hansa Center. (2014, July 2). Post Traumatic Stress Disorder: Healing the Wounds. Retrieved from http://www.davidjernigan.blogspot.com.

CHAPTER 14: DEPRESSION

Cited References:

1. McGill University (2007, October 24). *Cannabis: Potent Antidepressant In Low Doses Worsens Depression At High Doses.* Science Daily. Retrieved April 29, 2011, from http://www.sciencedaily.com/releases/2007/10/071023183937.ht

Other references for this chapter:

• Woollaston, V. (2013, August 22). *Could marijuana be GOOD for mental health? Breakthrough study claims the drug could be used to help treat depression.* Retrieved September 20, 2014, from http://www.dailymail.co.uk/sciencetech/article-2400032/Could-marijuana-GOOD-mental-health-Breakthrough-study-claims-drug-used-help-treat-depression.html

• MedicalMarijuana.com. (2011, April 29). *Medical Marijuana as a Treatment for Depression.* Retrieved October 9, 2014, from http://medicalmarijuana.com/experts/expert/title.cfm?artID=65

• Bambico, F., Katz, N., Debonnel, G., & Gobbi, G. (2007). Cannabinoids Elicit Antidepressant-Like Behavior and Activate Serotonergic Neurons through the Medial Prefrontal Cortex. *The Journal of Neuroscience, 27*(43), 11700-11711.

• Strasheim, C. (n.d.). Lyme Bytes. Retrieved December 1, 2014, from http://lymebytes.blogspot.com/2011/05/highlights-from-deep-look-beyond-lyme.html

- Whitlock Kelli. "Casting Prozac upon the waters." *University of Georgia Research Magazine,* Summer 2005.

- P. Andrews et. al., *"Primum non nocere:* An evolutionary analysis of whether antidepressants do more harm than good"

- Ramon Pelagio-Flores et al., "Serotonin, a tryptophan-derived signal conserved in plants and animals, regulates root system architecture probably acting as a neural auxin inhibitor in Arabidopsis thaliana," 490

CHAPTER 15: ANXIETY

Cited References:

1. Orta, G. (1563). *Colloquies on the Simples and Drugs of India.* Goa: Johannes de Endem.

2. Innes, E. (2014, March 7). Cannabis CAN reduce anxiety levels—but only in small doses. Retrieved October 12, 2014, from http://www.dailymail.co.uk/health/article-2575646/ Cannabis-CAN-reduce-anxiety-levels-say-doctors-small-doses.htm

3. Action of cannabidiol on the anxiety and other effects produced by delta 9-THC in normal subjects. *Psychopharmacology (Berl).* 76(3):245-50. PubMed PMID: 6285406

4. Bergamaschi M., et al. (2011). Cannabidiol Reduces the Anxiety Induced by Simulated Public Speaking in Treatment-Naive Social Phobia Patients. *Neuropsychopharmacology,36*(6), 1219-1226. Published online Feb 9, 2011. doi: 10.1038/npp.2011.6

5. Zuardi AW, Shirakawa I, Finkelfarb E, Karniol IG. (1982).

Other references for this chapter:

- TruthOnPot. (2013, May 23). *Can Marijuana Treat Anxiety Disorders?* Retrieved October 14, 2014, from http://www.truthonpot.com/2013/05/23/can-medical-marijuana-treat-anxiety-disorders/

- Christensen R, Kristensen PK, Bartels EM, Bliddal H, Astrup A. (2007 Nov 17). Efficacy and safety of the weight-loss drug rimonabant: a meta-analysis of randomised trials. Lancet. 370(9600):1706-13. Review. Erratum in: Lancet. 2008 Feb 16;371(9612):558. PubMed PMID: 18022033.

CHAPTER 16: SEIZURES AND CONVULSIONS

Cited References:

1. Bud, M. (2013, August 19). *Dr. O'Shaughnessy: Cannabis Was Medicine Before Prohibition.* Retrieved October 17, 2014, from http://marijuana.com/news/2013/08/

dr-oshaughnessy-cannabis-was-medicine-before-prohibition/

2. Hill D., T., Cascio G., M., & Romano, B., et. al (2013). Cannabidivarin-rich cannabis extracts are anticonvulsant in mouse and rat via a CB1 receptor-independent mechanism. British Journal of Pharmacology, 170(3), 679-92. Retrieved October 17, 2014, from http://www.ncbi.nlm.nih.gov/pubmed/23902406

Other references for this chapter:

- Jan. (n.d.). *Epilepsy/Seizure Disorder.* Retrieved October 16, 2014, from http://medicalmarijuana.com/medical-marijuana-treatments/Epilepsy/Seizure-Disorder

- Jan. (n.d.). *Epilepsy—Can Medical Marijuana Aid in Relieving Seizures?* Retrieved October 16, 2014, from http://medicalmarijuana.com/experts/expert/title.cfm?artID=75

- Bazian. (2014, May 23). *Could a compound found in cannabis treat epilepsy?* (NHS Choices, Ed.). Retrieved October 17, 2014, from http://www.nhs.uk/news/2014/05May/Pages/Could-a-compound-found-in-cannabis-treat-epilepsy.aspx

- Devinsky, O., Cilio, M.R., Cross, H., et. al (2014). Cannabidiol: Pharmacology and potential therapeutic role in epilepsy and other neuropsychiatric disorders. Epilepsia, 55(6), 791-802.

CHAPTER 17: RAGE

Cited References:

1. Jan. (2014, January 1). Limbic Rage Syndrome. Retrieved October 18, 2014, from http://medicalmarijuana.com/ medical-marijuana-treatments/Limbic-Rage-Syndrome

Other references for this chapter:

- *Chronic Co-infections of Lyme Disease—Symptoms of untreated co infections.* (2014, March 1). Retrieved October 19, 2014, from http://www.lyme-symptoms.com/ ChronicCoInfectionSymptoms.htm

- Sponaugle, M. (2012, January 1). *Lyme Disease Treatment | Sponaugle Wellness Institute.* Retrieved October 19, 2014, from http://sponauglewellness.com/

- Spiegel, J. (2013, March 11). *Medical Marijuana for Psychiatric Disorders.* Retrieved October 19, 2014, from http://www.psychologytoday. com/blog/mind-tapas/201303/ medical-marijuana-psychiatric-disorders

- *Marijuana for Depression and Bipolar Disorder.* Retrieved October 17, 2014, from http://patients4medicalmarijuana. wordpress.com/medical-use-of-cannabis-video/ marijuana-for-depression-bipolar/

- Ashton, C., Moore, P., & Et. al. (2005). Cannabinoids in bipolar affective disorder: A review and discussion of their

therapeutic potential. Journal of Psychopharmacology
19(3), 293-300.

CHAPTER 18: STRESS

Cited references:

1. Abush, H., & Akirav, I. (2013). Cannabinoids
    Ameliorate Impairments Induced by Chronic Stress
    to Synaptic Plasticity and Short-Term Memory.
    Neuropsychopharmacology, 2013(38), 1521-1534.

2. Zoppi, S., Nievas, B., Madrigal, J., Manzanares, J., Leza, J., &
    García-Bueno, B. (2010). Regulatory Role of Cannabinoid
    Receptor 1 in Stress-Induced Excitotoxicity and
    Neuroinflammation. Neuropsychopharmacology, 36(4),
    805-818.

Other references for this chapter:

*   Adams, M. (2014, February 25). *How Marijuana Fights
    Chronic Stress-Related Diseases.* Retrieved October
    21, 2014, from http://www.hightimes.com/read/
    how-marijuana-fights-chronic-stress-related-diseases

*   Gunduz-Cinar, O., Hill, M., Mcewen, B., & Holmes, A. (2013).
    Amygdala FAAH and anandamide: Mediating protection and
    recovery from stress. *Trends in Pharmacological Sciences,
    34*(11), 637-644.

- Dlugos, A., Childs, E., Stuhr, K., Hillard, C., & Wit, H. (2012). Acute Stress Increases Circulating Anandamide and Other N-Acylethanolamines in Healthy Humans. *Neuropsychopharmacology, 37*(11), 2416-2427.

- Segev, A., Rubin, A.S., Abush, H., Richter-Levin, G., & Akirav, I. (2013). Cannabinoid Receptor Activation Prevents the Effects of Chronic Mild Stress on Emotional Learning and LTP in a Rat Model of Depression. *Neuropsychopharmacology, 39*(4), 919-933.

- Zoppi, S., Madrigal, J.L., & Caso, R.J., et. al (2014). Regulatory role of the cannabinoid CB2 receptor in stress-induced neuroinflammation in mice. *British Journal of Pharmacology, 171*(11), 2814-2826.

- *Study: Marijuana May Combat Stress-Related Illnesses—Leaf Science.* (2014, February 14). Retrieved October 22, 2014, from http://www.leafscience.com/2014/02/24/study-marijuana-may-combat-stress-related-illnesses/

- Cannabinoids May Protect Brain From Stress-Related Impairments—Leaf Science. (2013, October 28). Retrieved October 22, 2014, from http://www.leafscience.com/2013/10/28/cannabinoids-may-protect-brain-stress-related-impairments/

CHAPTER 19: ADHD

Cited references:

1. Loflin, M., Earleywine, M., Leo, J., & Hobkirk, A. (2013). Subtypes of Attention Deficit-Hyperactivity Disorder (ADHD) and Cannabis Use. *Substance Use & Misuse, 49*(4), 427-34

2. Centonze, D., Bari, M., Di Michele, B., et. al (2009). Altered Anandamide Degradation In Attention-Deficit/ Hyperactivity Disorder.Neurology, 72(17), 1526-1527.

Other references for this chapter:

• Lu, A., Ogdie, M., Järvelin, M., et. al (2008). Association of the cannabinoid receptor gene (CNR1) with ADHD and post-traumatic stress disorder. *American Journal of Medical Genetics Part B: Neuropsychiatric Genetics,* 147B(8), 1488-1494.

• Mao, K. (2013, April 11). *Can Medical Cannabis Stop The ADHD Epidemic?—Waking Times «* *Waking Times.* Retrieved October 22, 2014, from http://www.wakingtimes.com/2013/04/11/ can-medical-cannabis-stop-the-adhd-epidemic/

• *Marijuana and ADHD: The Facts.* (2013, April 1). Retrieved October 22, 2014, from http://www.truthonpot. com/2013/04/01/medical-marijuana-and-adhd-the-facts/

• Miller, K., & Goldstein MD, E.T. (2013, August 6). *ASK Dr. G: Does Cannabis help Attention Deficit Disorder with Hyperactivity* (. Retrieved October 22, 2014, from http://normlwomensalliance.org/2013/08/06/ask-dr-g-does-cannabis-help-attention-deficit-disorder-with-hyperactivity-adhd/

• Olière, S., Joliette-Riopel, A., Potvin, S., & Jutras-Aswad, D. (2013). Modulation of the Endocannabinoid System: Vulnerability Factor and New Treatment Target for Stimulant Addiction. *Frontiers in Psychiatry, 4*(109).

• Marijuana May Treat Stimulant Addiction. (2013, December 24). Retrieved June 1, 2014.

CHAPTER 20: PSYCHOSIS/ SCHIZOPHRENIA-LIKE SYMPTOMS:

Cited References:

1. Moreau JJ (1845). *Du Hachisch et de l'Alienation Mentale: Etudes Psychologiques.* Librarie de Fortin Mason, Paris, France (English edition: Raven Press, New York, 1972).

2. Koethe, D., Giuffrida, A., Schreiber, D., Hellmich, M., Schultze-Lutter, F., et. al (2009). Anandamide elevation in cerebrospinal fluid in initial prodromal states of psychosis. *The British Journal of Psychiatry, 194*(4), 371-372.

3. Leweke, F., Piomelli, D., Pahlisch, F., et. al (2012). Cannabidiol enhances anandamide signaling and alleviates psychotic symptoms of schizophrenia. *Translational*

Psychiatry, 2012(2), E94-E94. Retrieved October 22, 2014, from

Other references for this chapter:

- Zuardi, A., Crippa, J., Hallak, J., et. al(2006). Cannabidiol, A Cannabis Sativa Constituent, As An Antipsychotic Drug. *Brazilian Journal of Medical and Biological Research,* 39(4), 421-29.

- Fergusson, D., Poulton, R., Smith, P., & Boden, J. (2006). Cannabis and psychosis. *BMJ,*332(7534), 172-175.

- *Chemicals in Cannabis may help mentally ill.* (2005, June 6). Retrieved October 22, 2014, from http://www.news-medical.net/news/2005/06/06/10716.aspx

- Chaturvedi, K. (2004). Cannabis as a psychotropic medication. *The British Journal of Psychiatry, 185*(78), 78-78

- *Cannabis does not induce schizophrenia, Dutch scientists say.* (2004, August 19). Retrieved October 20, 2014, from http://www.medicalnewstoday.com/releases/12283.php

- D'Souza DC, Perry E., MacDougall L., et. al (2004). The psychotomimetic effects of intravenous delta-9-tetrahydrocannabinol in healthy individuals: Implications for psychosis. Neuropsychopharmacology. 29: 1558-1572.

CHAPTER 21: NAUSEA AND VOMITING

- *Medical Cannabis: Research/Development and Clinical Trials—Vomiting-Documents.* (2014, January 1). Retrieved November 1, 2014, from http://www.unitedpatientsgroup. com/PatientsRoom-Nausea-Vomiting-Documents

- *Is Marijuana an Effective Treatment for Reducing Nausea and Vomiting from Chemotherapy?* (2010, July 12) Retrieved November 1, 2014 from http://medicalmarijuana.procon. org/view.answers.php?questionID=000137

- Abrahamov, A., Abrahamov, A., & Mechoulam, R. (1995). An efficient new cannabinoid antiemetic in pediatric oncology. *Life Sciences, 56*(23-24), 2097-2102.

- truthonpot.com. (2013, April 27). *Can Marijuana Cure Nausea?* Retrieved November 2, 2014 from http://www. truthonpot.com/2013/04/27/can-marijuana-cure-nausea/

- Goodin, S. (2002). 5-HT3-Receptor Antagonists for the Treatment of Nausea and Vomiting: A Reappraisal of Their Side-Effect Profile. *The Oncologist, 1*(2), 424-436.

- Parker, L., Rock, E., & Limebeer, C. (2011). Regulation of nausea and vomiting by cannabinoids. British Journal of Pharmacology, 163(7), 1411-1422.

CHAPTER 22: CACHEXIA OR WASTING SYNDROME

- Tazi, E., & Errihani, H. (2010). Treatment of cachexia in oncology. *Indian Journal of Palliative Care, 16*(3), 129-137.

- *Cachexia.* (2011). Retrieved November 1, 2014, from http://medicalmarijuana.com/medical-marijuana-treatments/Cachexia

- Strasser, F., Luftner, D., & Possinger, K., et. al (2006). Comparison Of Orally Administered Cannabis Extract And Delta-9-Tetrahydrocannabinol In Treating Patients With Cancer-Related Anorexia-Cachexia Syndrome: A Multicenter, Phase III, Randomized, Double-Blind, Placebo-Controlled Clinical Trial From The Cannabi. *Journal of Clinical Oncology,24*(21), 3394-3400.

- Aquino, G. (2005). Medicinal Marijuana: A Legitimate Appetite Stimulant? Nutrition Bytes,10(1).

CHAPTER 23: FINAL CONCLUSIONS ABOUT CANNABIS, THE INTELLIGENCE OF PLANTS, AND BACTERIA'S ELUSIVE ROLE IN EVOLUTION

Cited references:

1. Pollan, M. (2013, December 23). The Intelligent Plant—The New Yorker. Retrieved October 30, 2014, from http://www.newyorker.com/magazine/2013/12/23/the-intelligent-plant

2. Science Friday. (2014, January 10). *New research on plant intelligence may forever change how you think about plants.* Retrieved October 30, 2014, from http://www.pri.org/stories/2014-01-09/new-research-plant-intelligence-may-forever-change-how-you-think-about-plants

3. Buhner, S.H. (2013, November 20). The Doors of Perception and Belief Patterns. Retrieved from https://www.youtube.com/

Appendix

ANECDOTAL EXPERIENCES & SUCCESS STORIES

Alexis Kiri

My eyes started to blur as I proofread my work for the eighth time. On the morning of June 6, 2008, I was feverishly completing a midterm research paper for my Modern Philosophy class. I suddenly felt a horrific slicing sensation as if a blender was shredding my left arm. I stared at the throbbing limb. It was so painful that I expected it to be bleeding; yet it appeared to be in perfectly fine condition. No attack, no implosion, just my nerves firing out of control, and me helpless to fight back. From that moment, my perception of "normal" changed completely.

After almost two years of searching, I was diagnosed with fibro-myalgia and multiple joint pain. When I was only twenty, a rheu-matologist looked me in the eye and insisted, "You need to learn to deal with the pain because it is going to be like this forever. You can focus on maintaining a perfect diet and sleep schedule, and, with exercise, you might see little improvement. But don't hold your breath."

That wasn't good enough. To me, pain is just a signal to a prob-lem, not a diagnosis. I wouldn't stop looking that easily. It took seven specialists and eleven trips to the emergency room before anyone could identify my true diagnosis. Today, I know that I suffer from Late Stage Lyme disease.

On average, most Lyme patients go undiagnosed for five years. It is a cryptic condition. It wasn't until I suffered from symptoms in almost every system of my body that someone could put a name to it. My doctor explained that my disease is under wide debate in the medical community. The Center for Disease Control does not even *recognize* the chronic form.

This is *not* a conclusion that a deathly ill person wants to hear.

Usually, being diagnosed sheds light. Not for a Lyme patient. For me, having Lyme Disease is like being locked in a huge room packed tightly with sharp-edged furniture and china and glass, but without light, without windows or doors, and wearing a blindfold. I can't move without hurting myself, and I can't even see how I'm being hurt. Too little is known about the disease and its symptoms. . . .

My road to recovery has been as unique as my dental records. The experience is different for every Lyme patient; the symptoms present head-to-toe. Yet most of the victims manage to maintain normal lives, hiding our painful truth behind our pride. A large percentage of us, myself included, look healthy to the naked eye. But I know and feel my curse too intimately to ever be fooled.

Pain is an enigma. Our nerves are evolutionarily programmed to warn us of danger, of a problem in need of attention, but Lyme tricks the nerves into panic mode. I endure a litany of false alarms, and must distinguish *when* to listen *intellectually* rather than naturally.

The pain in my left arm spread first to my right, then down my back and into my legs. I cannot sit in a chair or ride in a car for more than a half hour on a good day without experiencing severe discomfort in my legs and hips. I have developed circulation problems, muscle spasms, ocular migraines, nausea, light sensitivity, head pressure, depersonalization and fatigue. Sometimes I make cognitive errors in speech, and I suffer random anemic fainting spells. I won't pretend these symptoms don't frighten me, but, over time, they have simply become part of my new paradigm, a lifestyle that has been forced upon me rather than chosen.

Living in chronic pain is a commitment to battle. I have to fight for happiness, and for freedom. I have struggled to establish my particular, even alien, lifestyle. I initially devoted myself to this raging war and lost the first battle; several months of intravenous antibiotics left my digestive tract in ruins. The day after Christmas 2010, I was rushed to the hospital to be diagnosed with hemorrhagic colitis. I was taken off antibiotics. Since then, I've endured a colonoscopy and two endoscopies to diagnose me with gastritis, polyps, esophagitis, and a hiatal hernia.

I was only 23 years old.

In June of 2011, I was diagnosed with numerous allergies including wheat, dairy, eggs, and tuna. Thus, I lost 25% of my body weight that year. I am 5'2" and I weigh 90 pounds if I consume, on average, 2,000 calories a day. The incessant nausea I experience usually permits only that much.

My intense suffering has made me desperate for a solution.

I have altered and adjusted my dreams and desires to work around my limitations. My pain controls my freedom. I have been prescribed hydrocodone, oxycodone, lorazepam, and cyclobenzaprine. These narcotics changed my mood and personality, and did *nothing* to relieve the relentless nerve pain.

My only relief stems from *cannabis*, but I am desperate for a more permanent solution to the problem. In the hospital, I have needed to have morphine or lorazepam through an IV to accomplish what smoking two grams of *cannabis* does on the comfort of my couch, in a fraction of the time.

I understand the importance of peace in my bones.

Medical *cannabis* gives me tranquility. The escape from pain that it provides keeps me sane. It allows me to combat the nausea and keep my weight above dangerous levels. With its help, I can eat, sleep, use my arms, and even stop my muscle spasms and migraines.

I finally found a team of doctors in California that could hear the word *cannabis* and not flinch but, instead, understand it as an essential part of my pain management protocol and still focus on the big picture.

As the years pass, my treatment evolves from one supplement to another, but a couple of themes remain constant in my life independently:*cannabis* and my team of doctors. Not that my doctors had a problem with it, but it was something which they didn't advise specifically.

One day, someone at a medical marijuana event brought up the idea of juicing *cannabis*. It sounded like another one of those green juice fads that I had no interest in trying. I was a meat and potatoes kind of gal who only liked my veggies steamed and with butter. No matter what homeopathic remedy I tried, my nutritionist kept coming back to the green smoothie, sure that I needed to give it a try.

I finally agreed, determined to give it a fair shot. I drove to Whole Foods and ordered my first Green Machine: 12oz of spinach, celery, carrot, parsley, cucumber, and coconut water. The taste was putrid; I gagged, certain that this was by far the most vile drink I had ever consumed. The beverage tasted like it came from a bottomless well, a witch's cauldron. My doctor said, "Your taste buds will change... it's important not to drink or eat anything after and let the flavor sit in your mouth." It was hard to believe him ...at first.

Within two weeks, I was ordering the 16oz Green Machine, guzzling the dark green liquid down within ten minutes. The sweetness of the carrot had started to taste like candy, the robust flavor a subconscious code for instant energy. I had transformed into a green juice enthusiast.

When I realized that these smoothies could include *cannabis* as part of my greens, I decided, one morning, to throw a few fresh leaves in my smoothie. My partner, Aaron, and I had been growing since moving out to California from Florida in 2011.

The leaves on the plants were being wasted; we had no access to a compost, living, as we did, in a tiny apartment. These leaves are thrown in composts and yard waste piles by the pound all over the world when they are rich in omegas, protein, and hold non-psychoactive cannabinoid acids that I wanted to start consuming, instead of losing. I upgraded my blender and began supplementing my daily smoothies with *cannabis*, in addition to spinach, and immediately felt like the healthiest me I ever remembered.

In 2008, at the beginning of this story, the Alexis born to my parents died. And I was reborn in pain, my stars rewritten by microscopic spirochetes. Juicing *cannabis* is my peaceful protest. It has allowed me to relearn how, not simply to survive, but to *live* with chronic pain. I understand that having complete control was always a figment of my imagination, but that doesn't mean I must relinquish my fate to the tiny bacteria that have invaded my body. This is a fight I'm now determined to win, because I have finally found the right tools.

My energy levels are up; my days are now increasingly pain-free. Access to live cannabis plants has been my secret. I want to impart that, while it can be a daunting quest to heal the human body, there is hope to be found.

Even in something as unexpected as a flower.

For more of Alexis's story, look for her book, coming out next Fall.

Francesca S

It seems almost funny to me now...that I didn't know when I was a teenager that I already had Lyme Disease, and I also didn't know that I was medicating with cannabis, the very herb I was told was so bad for my health and wellbeing. But of course it isn't funny. It is incredibly sad. Twenty years later I am finally aware of why I have struggled with my health, terribly so in the last six years, and why the ongoing use of cannabis could have saved me an immense amount of nearly unbearable pain over the years.

In my early twenties, I stopped using cannabis entirely. A decade later, when I first realized cannabis might help me with pain, I tried to use it again but it seemed to exacerbate my symptoms. It wasn't until years later when I found out I had Lyme and discovered Shelley's work that I first understood that returning to cannabis use had initially been causing me herxheimer reactions that I just needed to wait out. Once I knew that, and that medicating with an oil (I use cannabis-infused coconut oil) was the best method, I began to explore in earnest. Learning what Shelley presented about cannabis as a treatment for Lyme and associated coinfections and symptoms gave me incredible hope in a painfully challenging time.

I first tried CBD pills and quickly discovered that they were the most potent natural anti-inflammatory product I had ever tried—and I had tried *everything,* sometimes taking up to five high-quality natural anti-inflammatory products at a time. It's too bad that it wasn't enough, and for many years I resorted to 1000mg of Ibuprofen in order to sleep at night. I knew it was harming my stomach and gut lining and ultimately perpetuating my pain, but *nothing* else worked. If only I had known about the potent power of cannabis then.

Next, I tried vaporizing minute amounts (only one puff at a time) and experienced a reduction in pain, mood support, increased endurance, and better mental clarity. Then, just two weeks ago I began using the oil, starting again with a tiny dose (1/16th of a teaspoon) and gently working my way up (I am now at 1/8th teaspoon, sometimes twice a day). The change is powerful. In just two weeks I have noticed further reduction of pain, and improvements in mood, endurance, and sleep quality. I can only imagine the amount of other improvements I will see over time as I continue to use cannabis oil and increase my dose.

While to someone who has not known such pain, to simply say that cannabis helps in the ways I have described may seem minor, for someone who has lived with pain and dysfunction as severe as mine having relief like this feels like finding water in the desert...it feels as important as suddenly being able to breathe again when you have been suffocating. I knew when I was younger that this plant was my friend, and now I know it in a way that brings tears to my eyes. I couldn't be more appreciative for the healing power of this plant and medicine, and for Shelley and the life-changing information in this book. I will be forever grateful beyond all words.

SW

After four years of fighting a debilitating case of Lyme disease through antibiotics and various herbal remedies, I was still having symptoms that affected my everyday life which previous treatments did not help. I began to read positive results about using cannabis oil for Lyme disease. So, I decided to begin taking it myself last June. I basically took it 24 hours a day, taking one large dose before bed at night and smaller doses throughout the day so I could still function and fulfill any obligations. I did this for six months, and I stopped taking all other medicinal herbs during that time. It was the best six months I have experienced in years. I actually felt relatively normal again for the first time in a long time when I was taking cannabis oil, although it did not completely get rid of all of my symptoms. I still had mild symptoms of Bartonella and adrenal fatigue while taking it, they were just mild though.

Even though it felt like cannabis oil played a key role in giving me my life back, I started to get really nervous about accessing it because cannabis is illegal where I live. I had so much anxiety over the issue that, by the end of December, I decided that consistently getting enough to take it on a daily basis just wasn't worth the risk anymore. Since then, I have only been taking it before bed to help me get a good night's rest because extreme insomnia is one of the many symptoms of Lyme disease that I have. When I decided to quit getting cannabis, I saved what oil I did have left for this reason. Since I only use it at night, it has lasted me awhile.

After cutting back on my daytime dose of cannabis oil, I started another herbal medication in the morning along with my normal dose of cannabis oil at bedtime. During the last couple of weeks, my Bartonella symptoms have been raging and are worse than they were before I quit my daytime dose of oil. I don't know if this is a Herxheimer Reaction from starting a new herb, or if it's the disease progressing from cutting back so much on the cannabis oil. All I can say is that while I was on cannabis full time, it was the best I've felt in years. It's definitely a must have with this disease.

Anne S.

I am thankful every day of my life that I discovered the medicinal benefits of cannabis. Being chronically ill for years was miserable. Learning how to put on a fake smile and say you are fine is daunting. I got Lyme disease 10 years ago and that quickly turned into a diagnosis of Multiple Sclerosis (MS). I was shocked. I was a very active healthy 27 year old single mom who lived an adventurous life. The onset of my illness was rapid and severe. When I got Lyme I saw a bulls-eye rash and ignored it. I thought it was a spider bite, as I was told Lyme disease did not exist in Oregon. A few months later I developed a headache and lost partial eyesight in my left eye. I ignored it until my eyesight still had not returned a week later. I went to Urgent Care and was told it was a Migraine. I was given an injection and told to relax. In 30 minutes it had not gotten better and I was sent up to Optometry. The Doctor looked in my eye and told me he was positive I had MS. I was floored, I thought MS meant you were in a wheelchair. I knew little about the disease, and was referred to a Neurologist and had an MRI. The Doctor said I most likely had MS and sent me on my way. Two months later my eyesight cleared up. I was relieved. A few days later I lost eyesight in my right eye and went back to the Neurologist. He did another MRI and found lesions on my eyes, brain, and spine. He then told me I had tested positive for Lyme disease, but insisted I could not catch it in Oregon. He said he would need to test again. It was positive once more, so we tested again and again. Repeatedly, I was told there was no Lyme disease in Oregon. Meanwhile, my symptoms continued to increase. I was losing feeling on my left side, my balance was off, and I had weird tingling and zapping sensations all over my body. It is so scary when you begin to have bizarre neurological symptoms. You start to realize your brain controls every part of your body, and that you could become paralyzed, lose the ability to talk, or, if it hit the part of your brain that controls breathing, you could die. I lived in constant fear of every new sensation that arose in my body. I was put on antidepressants, anxiety medication, pain relievers, and sleeping pills. Despite testing positive, I still could not get a diagnosis of Lyme disease.

I eventually accepted I had Multiple Sclerosis and started the Disease Modifying Drug Avonex. It is a chemo therapy injection. Side effects include flu like symptoms, headaches, and suicidal depression. I unfortunately got all of the side effects. They upped my antidepressant medications and wished me the best of luck.

It became clear Avonex was not working for me, and my primary care doctor was worried about my mental state. I decided it was time to find out if I really had Lyme disease or not. I could not find a local doctor who was knowledgeable on the issue, so I flew thousands of miles to the Lyme disease Capitol –Lyme, Connecticut. The Harvard neurologist I saw quickly diagnosed me with Lyme disease, and apologized for the ordeal I had to go through to receive a proper diagnosis. At the time, I had no idea Lyme was a political issue that I was now stuck in the middle of. When I returned home with my new diagnosis and a prescription for IV medications, my local doctor didn't agree with the diagnosis or treatment plan and kicked me out of his office. I quickly found a new neurologist who also believed I had MS, but was open to considering my Lyme diagnosis and the treatment plan that accompanied it. The IV antibiotics were very hard on me. I became allergic to them and suffered from hives for 2 months. My new neurologist suggested Cannabis for symptoms. It was a much better option than adding more prescription pills. She wrote me a prescription for medical marijuana, and I smoked as much as I could. It did help with my pain and anxiety, but I was still taking a lot of pills and still felt very sick.

The IV antibiotics did help me at the time. I had an MRI shortly after, and the 13 lesions I had in my brain and spine were gone. I thought it was over and attempted to move on with my life, and got married and had a baby. I still had a few symptoms, but they were endurable. A couple months after my youngest daughter was born, I had the worst MS flare I had ever had. I could not feel my legs at all. I was walking into walls while holding my baby, and I was in constant pain. I was back on medications for sleeping, pain, and anxiety, and once again began smoking cannabis to help manage my symptoms. I went back on antibiotic treatment for Lyme disease, and had some ups and downs throughout the course of treatment. After a few years, my stomach could no longer handle antibiotics. I was spending 2 hours a day vomiting. I had started to accept that I would be sick for the rest of my life, that I would always have Lyme disease, and symptoms of MS. I decided to take my doctor's advice and learn to live the best life I could manage to live, despite the constant pain I lived in.

Eventually, I met a practitioner who practiced alternative medicine and had a more open mind. She said all disease is from toxicity, and that my body would begin to heal itself if I corrected my nutrient imbalances and removed the toxins from my body. Though I did not believe her at the time, I chose to listen to what she said because I felt I had nothing left to lose. She started slowly cleaning up my diet, asking me to give up sugar and switch to a vegetarian diet. That was tough for me, as I had previously drank a can of coke with every meal and loved dipping my fried chicken in ranch dressing. On Thanksgiving Day in 2013, I drank my last soda and ate as much junk food as I could. After starting my new diet, my digestion issues began improving within a few months. My new doctor then told me I needed to quit taking toxic pharmaceutical drugs every day if I wanted to recover fully. I had taken pharmaceuticals every day for 8 years, and she wanted me to somehow just completely quit them. I said "no" to her request, and ignored the entire issue for a bit. However, my husband reminded me that listening to her advice in the past had paid off, and asked me to seriously consider her advice in regards to getting off pharmaceuticals, as I could not realistically take pills every day for the rest of my life if I wanted to lead a healthy life-style. This helped me to finally come to the realization that I had become physically and mentally addicted pharmaceutical drugs.

I sat down with my practitioner and told her I was scared and I needed something to reduce my pain levels and to help me sleep. I had heard of others using cannabis oil—the strong kind of oil with cannabis extracted using food grade alcohol—to help with pain and sleep problems, and began to wonder if it could help with mine was well. She was not familiar with cannabis as a medicine, and felt I didn't need it. She did, however, appreciate that it was a plant, and that my grower took special care to grow organic. She agreed it was a much better option than the toxic pharmaceutical pills I was taking. I did a big 10 day Master Cleanse and stopped the toxic pills, replacing them with Cannabis Oil.

My grower makes the oil and puts it in Capsules that I take before bed. After I began taking the oil, I found it worked great to relieve some of my most horrible symptoms. Insomnia had been one of my horrible symptoms, and after starting the oil I finally began sleeping through the night. My pain began to fade, and cannabis oil began restoring my hope for a brighter future. One day I saw a video of a Doctor with PPMS, which is a type of MS where patients progressively decline with no hope of remission. In her video, she discussed how despite seeing top MS specialists and taking all of the most highly recommended MS drugs, she continued to rapidly decline. So, she started to research how to use food as a medicine. She developed a nutrient dense Paleo diet, focusing on 9 cups of vegetables a day. She is now out of her wheelchair and biking 18 miles in a day. Her video resonated with me and I ordered the book "Practical Paleo" by Diane Sanfilippo BS,NC. The first thing I read in the book "Let food be thy medicine, and medicine be thy food," a quote by Hippocrates, really resonated with me. In the book, the author said "know this: We are not smarter than Nature. We cannot make food better than nature. We need to eat real, whole food—period." That spoke to me. I felt it summarized the same problematic issues we face when trusting drug companies. They are not smarter than Nature. They cannot make better medicine than nature. We need to eat real, whole food—period.

I embrace my new natural life. Everything I put in my body, including food, products, and medicine, are all natural now. My practitioner was right. Once I got all the toxins out I started to heal. I have been in remission for over one year now. You are what you put in your body, and I now only eat real organic food and take organic cannabis oil. Multiple Sclerosis is an Auto Immune Disease that attacks the brain and spine. I do believe my disease had a cause, such as environmental toxins, GMO foods, and an underlying Lyme disease infection. There is still so much to learn about cannabis oil and how it works. I believe it healed my neurological problems, and likely has anti-inflammatory and antibacterial properties capable of treating Lyme disease and Multiple Sclerosis.

MAF

I use cannabis to treat many of the ailments that Lyme disease and Lyme co-infections have given me. Three and a half years ago, I began having digestive issues and constant heart burn. The pain was excruciating, my chest felt like it was on fire yet freezing at the same time—a raw fire that was constant. It started with digestive issues and constant heartburn that lasted several months. I tried over the counter drugs like Advil and Tylenol, as well as strong pharmaceutical pain relievers like Percocet and Vicodin. However, nothing helped with the pain. I was extremely fatigued every day, and bed ridden for nearly 9 months. On a scale of 1-10, my pain level was 8-9 on most days. Eventually, I chose to step outside of conventional western medicine for answers; as none of the doctors I saw, including a so called "specialist," were able to figure out what was wrong with me.

I sought out alternative treatments and medicine, and finally found a Naturopathic Doctor who actually looked at my entire symptom picture rather than just isolated ailments. She looked at the 60 plus symptoms I had, and tested me for Lyme disease. My test came back CDC negative but band 23, which is the band that is specific to the protein found on the spirochete, was positive. So, I was diagnosed with Lyme disease and was told I had a long road to recovery ahead of me. I was both sad and elated to finally receive a diagnosis and have a doctor who believed me, as opposed to thinking it was "all in my head."

I had used cannabis in the past, but more for recreational reasons than medicinal ones. At the height of my illness, I tried smoking cannabis and it made me feel incredibly awful. I later found out that smoking releases a large amount of cannabinoids into the system at an extremely rapid rate, and the awful symptoms I had experienced when smoking in the past were due to bacterial die-off. At first, I didn't understand just how powerful cannabis is as an anti-bacterial, anti-viral, anti-fungal, and anti-parasitic agent.

After detoxing for months to prepare my body, I decided to give cannabis another try, except this time I chose to ingest cannabis oil rather than smoking. I started with a tiny amount, no bigger than the size of a pinpoint. I took it on a cracker, and within 35 minutes I experienced extreme relief from pain, anxiety, and swelling, and basically noticed an overall improvement in my well-being. As I continued to treat with oil, I did start to have Herxheimer Reactions in response to bacterial die-off. I then realized that sublingual method (putting the oil under the tongue) was not as harsh as putting the oil on a cracker or a piece of bread. When you ingest the oil with food, your liver metabolizes the THC and it can make it seven times more potent than when you smoke it or sublingually ingest it. I prefer the sublingual ingestion and will soon be trying cannabis oil suppositories made with coconut oil for the first time. After 2 months on the oil, a fog lifted and my mind, body, and soul started feeling more in balance. I had to work a lot on detoxing, and aided my liver with herbs and frequently used a sauna, but was able to gain some quality of life back with the aid of cannabis. One of my main symptoms, which was the searing pain in my chest, is almost non-existent now due to cannabis. One aspect of the medicinal uses of cannabis that I found to be very effective was the raw form of THCa. When THCa is heated up it turns into THC, which is psychoactive. THCa in raw form is non psychoactive, but has tremendous pain relieving properties. Alta California Botanicals is a company that makes a particular raw THCa tincture that for me relieved my pain almost instantaneously. A few other people I know have tried the same oil, and it relieved their pain as well. I learned that herbal medicine can and will take some time to work, as it needs to build up in one's system, so it's important to express patience while letting the body find balance.

For many, as it was for me at first, cannabis oil can be a really harsh treatment as it causes extreme die off. So, starting with a less potent form of cannabis therapy like tinctures is a great, gentler approach. Currently, I still have some health issues and am still on my journey to healing, but I would not be where I am today without cannabis. It has been a major tool in my arsenal to combat the infectious toxic state my body has been in for years. Where I am today would not be possible without the use of cannabis. I will most likely continue to use cannabis for the rest of my life. I'm becoming more and more convinced that many people who are seriously ill are suffering from a deficiency in naturally occurring endocannabinoids, not unlike deficiencies in any type of minerals or vitamins. The endocannabinoid system exists in our bodies for a reason, and it is always good to make sure all systems in the body are being kept in proper balance.

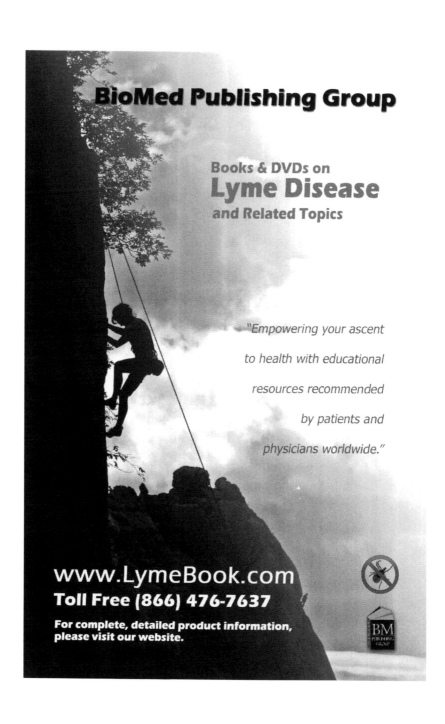

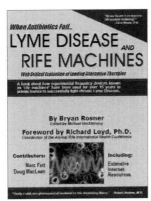

Book • $35

When Antibiotics Fail: Lyme Disease And Rife Machines, With Critical Evaluation Of Leading Alternative Therapies

By Bryan Rosner
Foreword by Richard Loyd, Ph.D.

There are enough books and websites about what Lyme disease is and which ticks carry it. But there is very little useful information for people who actually have a case of Lyme disease that is not responding to conventional antibiotic treatment. Lyme disease sufferers need to know their options, not how to identify a tick.

This book describes how experimental electromagnetic frequency devices known as rife machines have been used for over 15 years in private homes to fight Lyme disease. Also included are evaluations of more than 25 conventional and alternative Lyme disease therapies, including:

- Homeopathy
- IV and oral antibiotics
- Mercury detox.
- Hyperthermia / saunas
- Ozone and oxygen
- Samento®
- Colloidal Silver
- Bacterial die-off detox.

- Colostrum
- Magnesium supplementation
- Hyperbaric oxygen chamber (HBOC)
- ICHT Italian treatment
- Non-pharmaceutical antibiotics
- Exercise, diet and candida protocols
- Cyst-targeting antibiotics
- The Marshall Protocol®

Many Lyme disease sufferers have heard of rife machines, some have used them. But until now, there has not been a concise and organized source to explain how and why they have been used by Lyme patients. In fact, this is the first book ever published on this important topic.

The Foreword for the book is by Richard Loyd, Ph.D., coordinator of the annual Rife International Health Conference. The book takes a practical, down-to-earth approach which allows you to learn about*:

> "This book provides life-saving insights for Lyme disease patients."
>
> **- Richard Loyd, Ph.D.**

- Antibiotic treatment problems and shortcomings—why some people choose to use rife machines after other therapies fail.
- Hypothetical treatment schedules and sessions, based on the author's experience.
- The experimental machines with the longest track record: High Power Magnetic Pulser, EMEM Machine, Coil Machine, and AC Contact Machine.
- Explanation of the "herx reaction" and why it may indicate progress.
- The intriguing story that led to the use of rife machines to fight Lyme disease 20 years ago.
- Antibiotic categories and classifications, with pros and cons of each type of drug.
- Visit our website to read FREE EXCERPTS from the book!

*** Disclaimer:** Your treatment decisions must be made under the care of a licensed physician. Rife machines are not FDA approved and the FDA has not reviewed or approved of these books. The author is a layperson, not a doctor, and much of the content of these books is a statement of opinion based on the author's personal experience and research.*

Paperback book, 8.5 x 11", 203 pages, $35

The Top 10 Lyme Disease Treatments: Defeat Lyme Disease With The Best Of Conventional And Alternative Medicine

By Bryan Rosner
Foreword by James Schaller, M.D.

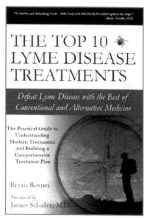

Book • $35

This information-packed book identifies ten promising conventional and alternative Lyme disease treatments and gives practical guidance on integrating them into a comprehensive treatment plan that you and your physician can customize for your individual situation and needs.

The book was not written to replace Bryan Rosner's first book (*Lyme Disease and Rife Machines*, opposing page). It was written to complement that book, offering Lyme sufferers many new foundational and supportive treatment options, based on the author's extensive research and years of personal experience. Topics include*:

- Systemic enzyme therapy, which helps detoxify tissues and blood, reduce inflammation, stimulate the immune system, and kill Lyme disease bacteria.
- Lithium orotate, a powerful yet all-natural mineral (belonging to the same mineral group as sodium and potassium) capable of profound neuroprotective activity.
- Thorough and extensive coverage of a complete Lyme disease detoxification program, including discussion of both liver and skin detoxification pathways. Specific detoxification therapies such as liver cleanses, bowel cleanses, the Shoemaker Neurotoxin Elimination Protocol, sauna therapy, mineral baths, mineral supplementation, milk thistle, and many others. Ideas to reduce and control herx reactions.
- Tips and clinical research from James Schaller, M.D.
- A detailed look at one method for utilizing antibiotics during a rife machine treatment campaign.
- Wide coverage of the Marshall Protocol, including an in-depth discussion of its mechanism of action in relation to Lyme disease pathology. Also, the author's personal experience with the Marshall Protocol over 3 years.
- An explanation of and new information about the Salt / Vitamin C protocol.
- Hot-off-the-press information on mangosteen fruit (not to be confused with mango) and its many benefits, including antibacterial, anti-inflammatory, and anti-cancer properties.
- New guidelines for combining all the therapies discussed in both of Rosner's books into a complete treatment plan. Brief and articulate for consideration by you and your doctor.
- Also includes updates on rife therapy, cutting-edge supplements, political challenges, an exclusive interview with Willy Burgdorfer, Ph.D. (discoverer of Lyme), and much more!

"Bryan Rosner thinks big and this new book offers big solutions."
- James Schaller, M.D.

"Another ground-breaking Lyme Disease book."
- Jeff Mittelman, moderator of the Lyme-and-rife group

"Brilliant and thorough."
- Nenah Sylver, Ph.D.

Do not miss this top Lyme disease resource. Discover new healing tools today!
Bring this book to your doctor's appointment to help with forming a treatment plan.

Paperback book, 7 x 10", 367 pages, $35

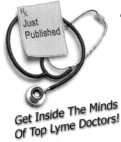
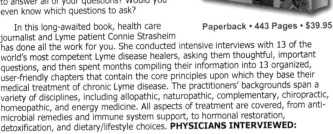
240

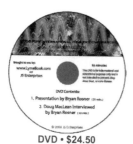

DVD • $24.50

Rife International Health Conference Feature-Length DVD (93 Minutes)

Bryan Rosner's Presentation and Interview with Doug MacLean

The Official Rife Technology Seminar Seattle, WA, USA

If you have been unable to attend the Rife International Health Conference, this DVD is your opportunity to watch two very important Lyme-related presentations from the event:

Presentation #1: Bryan Rosner's Sunday morning talk entitled *Lyme Disease: New Paradigms in Diagnosis and Treatment - the Myths, the Reality, and the Road Back to Health.* (51 minutes)

Presentation #2: Bryan Rosner's interview with Doug MacLean, in which Doug talked about his experiences with Lyme disease, including the incredible journey he undertook to invent the first modern rife machine used to fight Lyme disease. Although Doug's journey as a Lyme disease pioneer took place 20 years ago, this was the first time Doug has ever accepted an invitation to appear in public. This is the only video available where you can see Doug talk about what it was like to be the first person ever to use rife technology as a treatment for Lyme disease. Now you can see how it all began. Own this DVD and own a piece of history! (42 minutes)

Lymebook.com has secured a special licensing agreement with JS Enterprises, the Canadian producer of the Rife Conference videos, to bring this product to you at the special low price of $24.50. Total DVD viewing time: 1 hour, 33 minutes. We have DVDs in stock, shipped to you within 3 business days.

Price Comparison (should you get the DVD?)

Cost of attending the recent Rife Conference (2 people):
Hotel Room, 3 Nights = $400
Registration = $340
Food = $150
Airfare = $600
Total = $1,490

Cost of the DVD, which you can view as many times as you want, and show to family and friends:
DVD = $24.50

**Bryan Rosner
Presenting on
Sunday Morning
In Seattle**

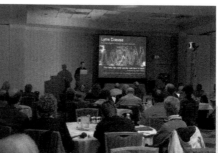

**DVD
93 Minutes
$24.50**

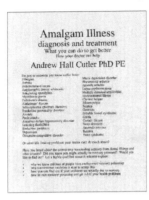

Amalgam Illness
diagnosis and treatment
What you can do to get better
How your doctor can help

Andrew Hall Cutler PhD PE

Book • $35

Amalgam Illness, Diagnosis and Treatment: What You Can Do to Get Better, How Your Doctor Can Help

By Andrew Cutler, PhD

This book was written by a chemical engineer who himself got mercury poisoning from his amalgam dental fillings. He found that there was no suitable educational material for either the patient or the physician. Knowing how much people can suffer from this condition, he wrote this book to help them get well. With a PhD in chemistry from Princeton University and extensive study in biochemistry and medicine, Andrew Cutler uses layman's terms to explain how people become mercury poisoned and what to do about it. The author's research shows that mercury poisoning can easily be cured at home with over-the-counter oral chelators – this book explains how.

In the book you will find practical guidance on how to tell if you really have chronic mercury poisoning or some other problem. Proper diagnostic procedures are provided so that sick people can decide what is wrong rather than trying random treatments. If mercury poisoning is your problem, the book tells you how to get the mercury out of your body, and how to feel good while you do that. The treatment section gives step-by-step directions to figure out exactly what mercury is doing to you and how to fix it.

"Dr. Cutler uses his background in chemistry to explain the safest approach to treat mercury poisoning. I am a physician and am personally using his protocol on myself."

- Melissa Myers, M.D.

Sections also explain how the scientific literature shows many people must be getting poisoned by their amalgam fillings, why such a regulatory blunder occurred, and how the debate between "mainstream" and "alternative" medicine makes it more difficult for you to get the medical help you need.

This down-to-earth book lets patients take care of themselves. It also lets doctors who are not familiar with chronic mercury intoxication treat it. The book is a practical guide to getting well. Sections from the book include:

• Why worry about mercury poisoning?
• What mercury does to you – symptoms, laboratory test irregularities, diagnostic checklist.
• How to treat mercury poisoning easily with oral chelators.
• Dealing with other metals including copper, arsenic, lead, cadmium.
• Dietary and supplement guidelines.
• Balancing hormones during the recovery process.
• How to feel good while you are chelating the metals out.
• How heavy metals cause infections to thrive in the body.
• Politics and mercury.

This is the world's most authoritative, accurate book on mercury poisoning.

Paperback book, 8.5 x 11", 226 pages, $35

Hair Test Interpretation: Finding Hidden Toxicities

By Andrew Cutler, PhD

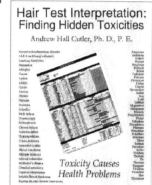

Hair Test Interpretation: Finding Hidden Toxicities

Andrew Hall Cutler, Ph. D., P. E.

Toxicity Causes Health Problems

Book • $35

Hair tests are worth doing because a surprising number of people diagnosed with incurable chronic health conditions actually turn out to have a heavy metal problem; quite often, mercury poisoning. Heavy metal problems can be corrected. Hair testing allows the underlying problem to be identified – and the chronic health condition often disappears with proper detoxification.

Hair Test Interpretation: Finding Hidden Toxicities is a practical book that explains how to interpret **Doctor's Data, Inc**. and **Great Plains Laboratory** hair tests. A step-by-step discussion is provided, with figures to illustrate the process and make it easy. The book gives examples using actual hair test results from real people.

One of the problems with hair testing is that both conventional and alternative health care providers do not know how to interpret these tests. Interpretation is not as simple as looking at the results and assuming that any mineral out of the reference range is a problem mineral.

Interpretation is complicated because heavy metal toxicity, especially mercury poisoning, interferes with mineral transport throughout the body. Ironically, if someone is mercury poisoned, hair test mercury is often low and other minerals may be elevated or take on unusual values. For example, mercury often causes retention of arsenic, antimony, tin, titanium, zirconium, and aluminum. An inexperienced health care provider may wrongfully assume that one of these other minerals is the culprit, when in reality mercury is the true toxicity.

> "This new book of Andrew's is the definitive guide in the confusing world of heavy metal poisoning diagnosis and treatment. I'm a practicing physician, 20 years now, specializing in detoxification programs for treatment of resistant conditions. It was fairly difficult to diagnose these heavy metal conditions before I met Andrew Cutler and developed a close relationship with him while reading his books. In this book I found his usual painful attention to detail gave a solid framework for understanding the complexity of mercury toxicity as well as the less common exposures. You really couldn't ask for a better reference book on a subject most researchers and physicians are still fumbling in the dark about."
> **- Dr. Rick Marschall**

So, as you can see, getting a hair test is only the first step. The second step is figuring out what the hair test means. Andrew Cutler, PhD, is a registered professional chemical engineer with years of experience in biochemical and healthcare research. This clear and concise book makes hair test interpretation easy, so that you know which toxicities are causing your health problems.

Paperback book, 8.5 x 11", 298 pages, $35

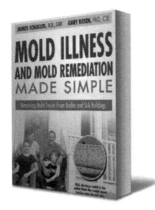

Book • $32.95

Mold Illness and Mold Remediation Made Simple: Removing Mold Toxins from Bodies and Sick Buildings

By James Schaller, M.D. and Gary Rosen, Ph.D.

Indoor mold toxins are much more dangerous and prevalent than most people realize. Visible mold in and around your house is far less dangerous than the mold you cannot see. Indoor mold toxicity, in addition to causing its own unique set of health problems and symptoms, also greatly contributes to the severity of most chronic illnesses.

In this book, a top physician and experienced contractor team up to help you quickly recover from indoor mold exposure. This book is easy to read with many color photographs and illustrations.

Paperback book, 8.5 x 11", 140 pages, $32.95
Also available on our website as an eBook!

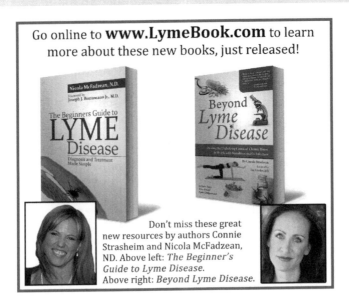

Go online to **www.LymeBook.com** to learn more about these new books, just released!

Don't miss these great new resources by authors Connie Strasheim and Nicola McFadzean, ND. Above left: *The Beginner's Guide to Lyme Disease.* Above right: *Beyond Lyme Disease.*

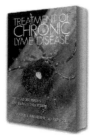

Treatment of Chronic Lyme Disease: 51 Case Reports and Essays In Their Regard

By Burton Waisbren Sr., MD, FACP, FIDSA

DON'T MISS THIS BOOK! A MUST-HAVE RESOURCE. What sets this Lyme disease book apart are the credentials of its author: he is not only a Fellow of the Infectious Diseases Society of America (IDSA), he is also one of its Founders! With 57+ years experience in medicine, Dr. Waisbren passionately argues for the validity of chronic Lyme disease and presents useful information about 51 cases of the disease which he has personally treated. His position is in stark contrast to that of the IDSA, which is a very powerful organization. **Quite possibly the most important book ever published on Lyme disease, as a result of the author's experience and credentials.**

Book • $24.95

Paperback book, 6x9", 169 pages, $24.95

Bartonella:
Diagnosis and Treatment

By James Schaller, M.D.

2 Book Set • $99.95

As an addition to his growing collection of informative books, Dr. James Schaller penned this excellent 2-part volume on Bartonella, a Lyme disease co-infection. The set is an ideal complementary resource to his Babesia textbook (next page).

Bartonella infections occur throughout the entire world, in cities, suburbs, and rural locations. It is found in fleas, dust mites, ticks, lice, flies, cat and dog saliva, and insect feces.

This 2-book set provides advanced treatment strategies as well as detailed diagnostic criteria, with dozens of full-color illustrations and photographs.

Both books in this 2-part set are included with your order.

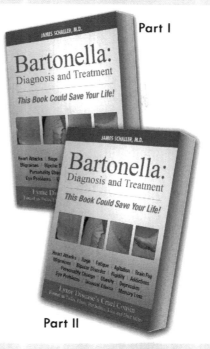

Part I

Part II

2 paperback books included, 7 x 10", 500 pages, $99.95

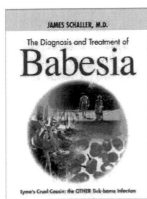

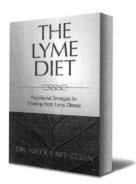

Book • $24.95

The Lyme Diet: Nutritional Strategies for Healing from Lyme Disease

By Nicola McFadzean, N.D.

We know about antibiotics and herbs. But what is the right diet for Lyme sufferers? Now you can read about the experience of Dr. Nicola McFadzean, N.D., in treating Lyme patients using proper diet.

The author is a Naturopathic Doctor and graduate of Bastyr University in Seattle, Washington. She is currently in private practice at her clinic, RestorMedicine, located in San Diego, California.

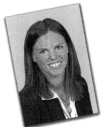

Nicola McFadzean, N.D.

This book covers numerous topics (not just diet-related):

- Reducing and controlling inflammation
- Maximizing immune function via dietary choices
- Restoring the gut & regaining healthy digestion
- Detoxification with food
- Hormone imbalances
- Biofilms
- Kefir vs. yogurt vs. probiotics
- Candida, liver support, and much more!

Paperback book, 6x9", 214 Pages, $24.95
Also available as an eBook on our website!

The Stealth Killer: Is Oral Spirochetosis the Missing Link in the Dental & Heart Disease Labyrinth? *By William D. Nordquist, BS, DMD, MS*

Can oral spirochete infections cause heart attacks? In today's cosmopolitan urban population, more than 51 percent of those with root canal–treated teeth probably have infection at the apex of their root. Dr. Nordquist, an oral surgeon practicing in Southern California, believes that any source of bacteria with resulting chronic infection (including periodontal disease) in the mouth may potentially lead to heart disease and other systemic diseases. With more than 40 illustrations and x-ray reproductions, this book takes you behind the scenes in Dr. Nordquist's research laboratory, and provides many tips on dealing with Lyme-related dental problems. A breakthrough book in dentistry & infectious disease!

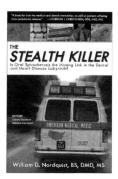

Paperback Book • $25.95

Paperback book, 6x9", 161 pages, $25.95

Rife's World of Electromedicine: The Story, the Corruption and the Promise

By Barry Lynes

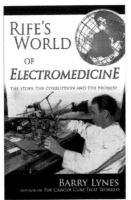

Book • $17.95

The cause of cancer was discovered in the early 1930's. It was a virus-sized, mini-bacteria or "particle" that induced cells to become malignant and grow into tumors. The cancer microbe or particle was given the name BX by the brilliant scientist who discovered it: Royal Raymond Rife.

Laboratory verification of the cause of cancer was done hundreds of times with mice in order to be absolutely certain. Five of America's most prominent physicians helped oversee clinical trials managed by a major university's medical school.

Sixteen cancer patients were brought by ambulance twice a week to the clinical trial location in La Jolla, California. There they were treated with a revolutionary electromedicine that painlessly, non-invasively destroyed only the cancer-causing microbe or particle named BX. After just three months of this therapy, all patients were diagnosed as clinically cured. Later, the therapy was suppressed and remains so today.

In 1987, Barry Lynes wrote the classic book on Rife history (*The Cancer Cure That Worked*, see catalog page 14). *Rife's World* is the sequel.

Paperback book, 5.5 x 8.5", 90 pages, $17.95

Physicians' Desk Reference (PDR) Books (opposing page)

Most people have heard of *Physicians' Desk Reference* (PDR) books because, for over 60 years, physicians and researchers have turned to PDR for the latest word on prescription drugs.

THOMSON™

You may not know that Thomson Healthcare, publisher of PDR, offers PDR reference books not only for drugs, but also for herbal and nutritional supplements. No available books come even close to the amount of information provided in these PDRs—*PDR for Herbal Medicines* weighs 5 lbs and has over 1300 pages, and *PDR for Nutritional Supplements* weighs over 3 lbs and has more than 800 pages.

> "I relied heavily on the PDRs during the research phase of writing my books. Without them, my projects would have greatly suffered."
>
> **- Bryan Rosner**

We carry all three PDRs. Although PDR books are typically used by physicians, we feel that these resources are also essential for people interested in or recovering from chronic disease. For the supplements, herbs, and drugs included in the books, you will find the following information: Pharmacology, description and method of action, available trade names and brands, indications and usage, research summaries, dosage options, history of use, pharmacokinetics, and much more! Worth the money for years of faithful use.

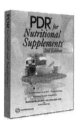

PDR for Nutritional Supplements *2nd Edition!*

This PDR focuses on the following types of supplements:

- Vitamins
- Minerals
- Amino acids
- Hormones
- Lipids
- Glyconutrients
- Probiotics
- Proteins
- Many more!

"In a part of the health field not known for its devotion to rigorous science, [this book] brings to the practitioner and the curious patient a wealth of hard facts."

- Roger Guillemin, M.D., Ph.D., Nobel Laureate in Physiology and Medicine

Book • $69.50

The book also suggests supplements that can help reduce prescription drug side effects, has full-color photographs of various popular commercial formulations (and contact information for the associated suppliers), and so much more! Become educated instead of guessing which supplements to take.

Hardcover book, 11 x 9.3", 800 pages, $69.50

PDR for Herbal Medicines *4th Edition!*

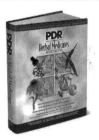

PDR for Herbal Medicines is very well organized and presents information on hundreds of common and uncommon herbs and herbal preparations. Indications and usage are examined with regard to homeopathy, Indian and Chinese medicine, and unproven (yet popular) applications.

In an area of healthcare so unstudied and vulnerable to hearsay and hype, this scientifically referenced book allows you to find out the real story behind the herbs lining the walls of your local health food store.

Use this reference before spending money on herbal products!

Book • $69.50

Hardcover book, 11 x 9.3", 1300 pages, $69.50

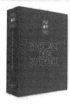

PDR for Prescription Drugs *Current Year's Edition!*

With more than 3,000 pages, this is the most comprehensive and respected book in the world on over 4,000 drugs. Drugs are indexed by both brand and generic name (in the same convenient index) and also by manufacturer and product category. This PDR provides usage information and warnings, drug interactions, plus a detailed, full-color directory with descriptions and cross references for the drugs. A new format allows dramatically improved readability and easier access to the information you need now.

Book • $99.50

Hardcover book, 12.5 x 9.5", 3533 pages, $99.50

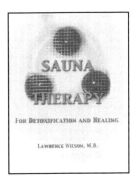

Book • $22.95

Sauna Therapy for Detoxification and Healing

By Lawrence Wilson, MD

This book provides a thorough yet articulate education on sauna therapy. It includes construction plans for a low-cost electric light sauna. The book is well referenced with an extensive bibliography.

Sauna therapy, especially with an electric light sauna, is one of the most powerful, safe and cost-effective methods of natural healing. It is especially important today due to extensive exposure to toxic metals and chemicals.

Fifteen chapters cover sauna benefits, physiological effects, protocols, cautions, healing reactions, and many other aspects of sauna therapy.

Dr. Wilson is an instructor of Biochemistry, Hair Mineral Analysis, Sauna Therapy and Jurisprudence at various colleges and universities including Yamuni Institute of the Healing Arts (Maurice, LA), University of Natural Medicine (Santa Fe, NM), Natural Healers Academy (Morristown, NJ), and Westbrook University (West Virginia). His books are used as textbooks at East-West School of Herbology and Ohio College of Natural Health. Go to www.LymeBook.com for free book excerpts!

Paperback book, 8.5 x 11", 167 pages, $22.95

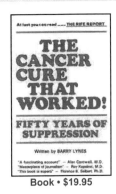

Book • $19.95

Over 50,000 Copies Sold!

The Cancer Cure That Worked: Fifty Years of Suppression

At Last You Can Read... The Rife Report

By Barry Lynes

Investigative journalism at its best. Barry Lynes takes readers on an exciting journey into the life work of Royal Rife. We are now the official publisher of this book. Call or visit us online for wholesale terms.

"A fascinating account..." -Alan Cantwell, MD

"This book is superb." -Florence B. Seibert, PhD

"Barry Lynes is one of the greatest health reporters in our country. With the assistance of John Crane, longtime friend and associate of Roy Rife, Barry has produced a masterpiece..." -Roy Kupsinel, M.D., editor of *Health Consciousness Journal*

Paperback book, 5 x 8", 169 pages, $19.95

Rife Video Documentary
2-DVD Set, Produced by
Zero Zero Two Productions

Must-Have DVD set for your Rife technology education!

In 1999, a stack of forgotten audio tapes was discovered. On the tapes were the voices of several people at the center of the events which are the subject of this documentary: a revolutionary treatment for cancer and a practical cure for infectious disease.

The audio tapes were over 40 years old. The voices on them had almost faded, nearly losing key details of perhaps the most important medical story of the 20th Century.

But due to the efforts of the Kinnaman Foundation, the faded tapes have been restored and the voices on them recovered. So now, even though the participants have all passed away...

...they can finally tell their story.

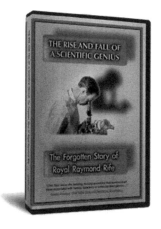

2-DVD Set • $39.95

"These videos are great. We show them at the Annual Rife International Health Conference."
-Richard Loyd, Ph.D.

"A mind-shifting experience for those of us indoctrinated with a conventional view of biology."
-Townsend Letter for Doctors and Patients

In the summer of 1934 at a special medical clinic in La Jolla, California, sixteen patients withering from terminal disease were given a new lease on life. It was the first controlled application of a new electronic treatment for cancer: the Beam Ray Machine.

Within ninety days all sixteen patients walked away from the clinic, signed-off by the attending doctors as cured.

What followed the incredible success of this revolutionary treatment was not a welcoming by the scientific community, but a sad tale of its ultimate suppression.

The Rise and Fall of a Scientific Genius documents the scientific ignorance, official corruption, and personal greed directed at the inventor of the Beam Ray Machine, Royal Raymond Rife, forcing him and his inventions out of the spotlight and into obscurity. **Just converted from VHS to DVD and completely updated.**

Includes bonus DVD with interviews and historical photographs! Produced in Canada.

Visit our website today to watch a FREE PREVIEW CLIP!

2 DVD-set, including bonus DVD, $39.95

251

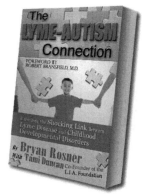

Book • $25.95

The Lyme-Autism Connection: Unveiling the Shocking Link Between Lyme Disease and Childhood Developmental Disorders

By Bryan Rosner & Tami Duncan

Did you know that Lyme disease may contribute to the onset of autism?

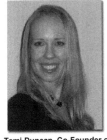

This book is an investigative report written by Bryan Rosner and Tami Duncan. Duncan is the co-founder of the *Lyme Induced Autism (LIA) Foundation*, and her son has an autism diagnosis.

Tami Duncan, Co-Founder of the Lyme Induced Autism (LIA) Foundation

Awareness of the Lyme-autism connection is spreading rapidly, among both parents and practitioners. *Medical Hypothesis*, a scientific, peer-reviewed journal published by Elsevier, recently released an influential study entitled *The Association Between Tick-Borne Infections, Lyme Borreliosis and Autism Spectrum Disorders*. Here is an excerpt from the study:

> "Chronic infectious diseases, including tick-borne infections such as Borrelia burgdorferi, may have direct effects, promote other infections, and create a weakened, sensitized and immunologically vulnerable state during fetal development and infancy, leading to increased vulnerability for developing autism spectrum disorders. An association between Lyme disease and other tick-borne infections and autistic symptoms has been noted by numerous clinicians and parents."

—Medical Hypothesis Journal.
Article Authors: Robert C. Bransfield, M.D., Jeffrey S. Wulfman, M.D., William T. Harvey, M.D., Anju I. Usman, M.D.

Nationwide, 1 out of 150 children are diagnosed with Autism Spectrum Disorder (ASD), and the LIA Foundation has discovered that many of these children test positive for Lyme disease/Borrelia related complex—yet most children in this scenario never receive appropriate medical attention. This book answers many difficult questions: How can infants contract Lyme disease if autism begins before birth, precluding the opportunity for a tick bite? Is there a statistical correlation between the incidences of Lyme disease and autism worldwide? Do autistic children respond to Lyme disease treatment? What does the medical community say about this connection? Do the mothers of affected children exhibit symptoms? **Find out in this book.**

Paperback book, 6x9", 287 pages, $25.95

Dietrich Klinghardt, M.D., Ph.D.
"Fundamental Teachings"
5-DVD Set

Includes Disc Exclusively For Lyme Disease!

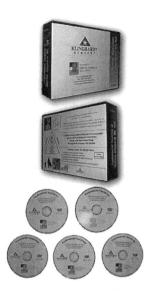

Dietrich Klinghardt, M.D., Ph.D. is a legendary healer known for discovering and refining many of the cutting-edge treatment protocols used for a variety of chronic health problems including Lyme disease, autism and mercury poisoning.

Now you can find out all about this doctor's treatment methods from the privacy of your own home! This 5-DVD set includes the following DVDs:

- **DISC 1**: The Five Levels of Healing and the Seven Factors

- **DISC 2**: Autonomic Response Testing and Demonstration

- **DISC 3**: Heavy Metal Toxicity and Neurotoxin Elimination / Electrosmog

- **DISC 4**: Lyme disease and Chronic Illness

- **DISC 5**: Psycho-Emotional Issues in Chronic Illness & Addressing Underlying Causes

5-DVD Set • $125

Dr. Dietrich Klinghardt is one of the most important contributors to modern integrative treatment for Lyme disease and related medical conditions. This comprehensive DVD set is a must-have addition to your educational library.

5-DVD Set, $125

Our catalog has space limitations, but our website does not! Visit www.LymeBook.com to see even more exciting products.

Don't Miss These New Books & DVDs, Available Online:
- Babesia Update 2009, by James Schaller, M.D.
- Marshall Protocol 5-DVD Set
- Cure Unknown, by Pamela Weintraub
- The Experts of Lyme Disease, by Sue Vogan
- The Lyme Disease Solution, by Ken Singleton, M.D.
- **Lots of Free Chapters and Excerpts Online!**

Don't use the internet? No problem, just call (530) 573-0190.

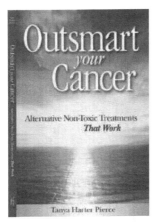

Outsmart Your Cancer:
Alternative Non-Toxic Treatments
That Work   By Tanya Harter Pierce

Why BLUDGEON cancer to death with common conventional treatments that can be toxic and harmful to your entire body?

When you OUTSMART your cancer, only the cancer cells die — NOT your healthy cells! *OUTSMART YOUR CANCER: Alternative Non-Toxic Treatments That Work* is an easy guide to successful non-toxic treatments for cancer that you can obtain right now! In it, you will read real-life stories of people who have completely recovered from their advanced or late-stage lung cancer, breast cancer, prostate cancer, kidney cancer, brain cancer, childhood leukemia, and other types of cancer using effective non-toxic approaches.

Book and Audio CD • $24.50

Plus, *OUTSMART YOUR CANCER* is one of the few books in print today that gives a complete description of the amazing formula called "Protocel," which has produced incredible cancer recoveries over the past 20 years. **A supporting audio CD is included with this book.** Pricing = $19.95 book + $5.00 CD.

Paperback book, 6 x 9", 437 pages, with audio CD, $24.95

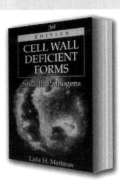

Cell Wall Deficient Forms: Stealth Pathogens

By Lida Mattman, Ph.D.

This is one of the most influential infectious disease textbook of the century. Dr. Mattman, who earned a Ph.D. in immunology from Yale University, describes her discovery that a certain type of pathogen lacking a cell wall is the root cause of many of today's "incurable" and mysterious chronic diseases. Dr. Mattman's research is the foundation of our current understanding of Lyme disease, and her work led to many of the Lyme protocols used today (such as the Marshall Protocol, as well as modern LLMD antibiotic treatment strategy). Color illustrations and meticulously referenced breakthrough principles cover the pages of this book. A must have for all serious students of chronic, elusive infectious disease.

Hardcover Book • $169.95

Hardcover book, 7.5 x 10.5", 416 pages, $169.95

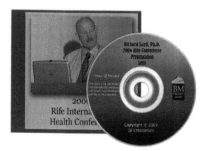

Richard Loyd, Ph.D., presents at the Rife International Health Conference in Seattle

Watch this DVD to gain a better understanding of the technical details of rife technology.

DVD • $24.50

Dr. Loyd, who earned a Ph.D. in nutrition, has researched and experimented with numerous electrotherapeutic devices, including the Rife/Bare unit, various EMEM machines, F-Scan, BioRay, magnetic pulsers, Doug Machine, and more. Dr. Loyd also has a wealth of knowledge in the use of herbs and supplements to support Rife electromagnetics.

By watching this DVD, you will discover the nuts and bolts of some very important, yet little known, principles of rife machine operation, including:

- Gating, sweeping, session time
- Square vs. sine wave
- DC vs. AC frequencies
- Duty cycle
- Octaves and scalar octaves

- Voltage variations and radio frequencies
- Explanation of the spark gap
- Contact vs. radiant mode
- Stainless vs. copper contacts
- A unique look at various frequency devices

DVD, 57 minutes, $24.50

Under Our Skin:
Lyme Disease Documentary Film

A gripping tale of microbes, medicine & money, UNDER OUR SKIN exposes the hidden story of Lyme disease, one of the most serious and controversial epidemics of our time. Each year, thousands go undiagnosed or misdiagnosed, often told that their symptoms are all in their head. Following the stories of patients and physicians fighting for their lives and livelihoods, the film brings into focus a haunting picture of the health care system and a medical establishment all too willing to put profits ahead of patients.

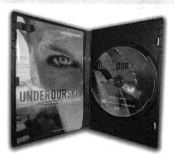

DVD • $34.95

Bonus Features: 32-page discussion guidebook, one hour of bonus footage, director's commentary, and much more! FOR HOME USE ONLY

DVD with bonus features, 104 minutes, $34.95 MUST SEE!

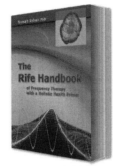